April, 2011

Christina,

This is my story from "before".
I think the essence (i.e. the love of
clinical work) shines through...
thankyou for everything in our
                              current work
        Together, Ildiko

SENSATIONS
THE HEALING POWER OF HOMEOPATHY

ILDIKO RAN, CCH
with
ANNA MENYHÉRT, PhD

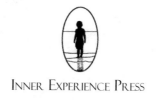

INNER EXPERIENCE PRESS

© Ildiko Ran, Anna Menyhért 2007

Inner Experience Press
19 Edmund Road, Arlington MA, 02474
www.innerexperience.com
(781) 775-1617
office@innerexperience.com

First Printing 2007
Library of Congress Control Number: 2007936119
ISBN 978-0-9799303-0-0
Printed in the United States of America
Printed by Data Reproductions Corporation

Cover design by Marx Fertik
Cover art by Sophie Glikson, MA, LMHC, CET (Title of the original piece: *Softening*)
Edited by Kevin Quirk
Typesetting by Anna Menyhért

Attention Corporations, Universities, Colleges, and Professional Organizations: Quantity Discounts are available on bulk purchases of this book for educational, gift purposes, or as premiums for increasing magazine subscriptions or renewals. For information please contact Inner Experience Press.

Please Note: This book is for educational purposes only. Although the authors and publishers have exhaustively researched all sources to ensure the accuracy and completeness of the information contained in this book, we assume no responsibility for errors, inaccuracies, omissions, or any inconsistency herein. Any slights of people or organizations are unintentional. This book is not intended to be used for self-diagnosis and self-treatment. Readers should use their own judgment and consult a homeopathic practitioner for specific applications to their individual problems.

ACKNOWLEDGEMENTS

First and most my gratitude goes towards my immediate family that has supported me throughout my career as a homeopath and more recently as an author. My husband, Alexander Ran, who was the first one to suggest that I should become a homeopath, when I was still reluctant, thinking this career would not suit me. How wrong I was! He is usually right in his predictions and I am forever grateful for that. Our wonderful children, Niva, Sonia, Yona, and Beni, who proudly tell their friends that their mom is a homeopath, and are well-prepared with their own explanation of homeopathy for all those who have no clue what it is. These are my children, who, at an early age, when playing doctors, did not listen to each other's chest with a stethoscope, but rolled up tissue paper into tiny white balls, and handed them out to each other as the promise of cure. Niva also helped me with her insightful remarks on the manuscript. Nomi, the youngest one gives inspiration to all of us with her charming presence. I want to thank Moshe Shulman and Yumi Thomas, who provided me with time, a most important component when writing a book. Thank you.

I am grateful to my fast and accurate editor, Kevin Quirk, who turned the manuscript into legible English and the best read it could be; Sophie Glikson, artist, and expressive arts therapist, who contributed the beautiful and sensational artwork for the cover; Cecile Rêve, for her help with graphic design; and Melleta Marx and Joshua Fertik of Marx Fertik Design for giving me a helping hand when I needed it.

Among homeopaths I want to acknowledge Ritva Laureaus, the first homeopath I ever met, who gave me the first books on homeopathy, which opened a new world for me; my teachers, who have been the cornerstones of my career as a homeopathic practitioner: the inspirational Ian Watson, Robin Murphy, Rajan Sankaran, Jo Daly, Misha Norland, Paul Herscu, Amy Rothenberg, Jeremy Sherr, and Jayesh Shah. I also want to extend my gratitude to Dr. Meghna Shah, the gateway of information to Dr. Sankaran's work, who whole-heartedly gives her time to maintain and expand the network of homeopaths who have been inspired by Dr. Sankaran's work.

I want to thank Judyth Reichenberg-Ullman, for her advice and praise of the manuscript, Julian Jonas, for his insights and for sharing the book with his students, Nicole Bacon for reading the manuscript from the point of view of a devoted yogini, and Dr. Gillian Katz Wies, reviewing it from yet another perspective. I am grateful to Amy Lansky, who gave me kind and genuine advice on starting the process of writing and publishing a book. She guided me towards Marylin and Tom Ross's book on self-publishing, who's advice I took almost step-by-step. Thank you all.

Ildiko Ran

CONTENTS

INTRODUCTION

PRELUDE

Homeopathy has always been a dynamic healing art. It has been evolving ever since its origins in the 1800s. Dr. Samuel Hahnemann, the founder of homeopathy, revised his *Organon of Medicine*, the book that covers the guiding principles of homeopathy, several times. He used his newly found medicine with success but he was driven to improve it until the end of his life. Many of his successors have been expanding on his ideas and the result is a vibrant healing art that utilizes the laws of nature, some of which were explained by modern science long after they had been used in homeopathic philosophy successfully. Even though homeopathy has been enhanced, its basic principles have not changed. These principles have been established in accordance with nature that is not affected by time.

The most recent development in homeopathy started in the 1990s, when Dr. Rajan Sankaran and his Bombay group of homeopathic doctors started working on a new approach, which since then has been called the Sensation Method. This method has created a shift in the practice of homeopathy. The book you are holding in your hands was born out of a growing interest among people who have been healed by homeopathy using the Sensation Method and practitioners seeking more efficient ways to help their clients.

Our present time is an exciting period to practice homeopathy as we feel we are a part of a historical, evolutionary process. The same can be said about our current time in human history. There are great challenges during times like these, just as there are great revelations. Successes achieved using the new way of thinking can be as exciting as witnessing a child first learn to walk. Just as parents proudly watch their offspring mastering their new skills, homeopaths take heart in seeing the results this new approach to homeopathy is capable of achieving. This process requires great skill and an open mind. Dr. Sankaran has made a great contribution through such books as *The Spirit of Homoeopathy* (1991), *The Substance of Homoeopathy* (1994), *The Soul of Remedies* (1997), *The System of Homoeopathy* (2000), *An Insight into Plants* (2002), *Sankaran's Schema* (2005), *The Sensation in Homoeopathy* (2004), *Sensation Refined* (2007), that convey his new findings and additions to the system. He persistently shares his ideas and discoveries with a broad spectrum of homeopathic practitioners worldwide. Nevertheless, there remains a need to bring this information in palatable ways to practitioners who still may not be familiar with the Sensation Method and to non-practitioners from the general public who may have only limited experience with homeopathy or who may be considering using it for the first time. I hope this book bridges that gap and can serve to bring the simple elegance of this method to a wider audience. The case studies included in this book were mainly influenced by this new way of thinking. I am truly grateful to Dr. Sankaran for the depth and beauty of healing that has been revealed through this method.

I had studied the works of renowned homeopathic masters and had been applying their insights in my practice, but once I started implementing the Sensation Method it became clear to me that the level of understanding of the human state had reached an entirely new level. That is why the main focus in my homeopathic practice has been this method. I trust that you will share my appreciation for the method and enjoy the unfolding of its depth. While I am indebted for the insights of Dr. Sankaran, I take full responsibility for all the shortcomings of the cases presented here. This book is the result of my own understanding and use of the method in practice. My aim is to share it with you, so that you may see the clarity, precision and grace in this system of healing and consider how it might benefit you in your own life.

AUTHOR'S NOTE

This book has been written to introduce the reader to a particular method used in homeopathy. If this is the first book on homeopathy that you hold in your hands I believe you will gain important insights and understanding of what the work of a homeopath, who works with the Sensation Method entails. Nevertheless if you would like to get a full picture of the history, practice and philosophy of the art and science of homeopathy I would refer you to some comprehensive books that have been written with that goal in mind. Please look for those titles in the Suggested Readings. It is important to emphasize that there are essential basic ideas in homeopathy the Sensation Method rests upon, which the scope of this book does not allow to explore.

The first chapter of this book is an introduction to homeopathy, with the main focus on the Sensation Method. It describes the system, the process, the tools, and the goal of treatment. The rest of the book is divided into three chapters based on the kingdom the remedies are derived from: mineral, plant, and animal. In each of those chapters, after an in-depth introduction to the respective kingdom characteristics you can read real, live cases, written up in a dialogue format. Explanations are included for easier understanding, and are distinguished by indented paragraphs. The homeopath's questions are italicized. All the cases emerged from my clinical experience. The essence and flow of the interviews have not been altered, although they have been abbreviated to make them easier to follow and understand. All personally identifying information and names have been changed to protect the privacy of my clients.

There are ten cases in the book, three of which were taken by Anna Menyhért, who has been my supervisee during this process. Ms. Menyhért lives and works in Hungary, so when reading those cases bear in mind the different environment from the cases taken in the United States. Ms. Menyhért also has been instrumental in the writing of this book. She first inspired me to start this project and, being a writer, she lent her expertise not only as an insightful homeopath but also in helping me to establish the structure of the book and the style of the cases.

When reading this book please remember that not all homeopaths apply the Sensation Method. When I describe the work and thinking process of a homeopath, I mean only those homeopaths that work with this method. On the other hand sometimes you might meet medical doctors, therapists and practitioners of various modalities that follow very similar ideas to the ones expressed in this book. Their tools are different, they might not even have heard of the Sensation Method, but the guiding principles they use are very similar to the ones described in this book. I believe that the more healing modalities find their way to the same source, it is a sign that we all understand something very meaningful, something very close to the vital core of humanity.

Boston, September 2007

Ildiko Ran

CHAPTER 1
NEED FOR A PARADIGM SHIFT

Descending from the thinking mind into the feeling body is a great challenge for many people, but it's a challenge that more and more people are taking these days. Body-mind therapies have been flourishing across the Western world in recent decades. Yoga, Reiki, Qigong, massage, essential oils used in spas, and other grounding exercises are on the rise. People of all ages have begun to recognize that for the mind to work at its best, the body needs nourishment. Nourishing the body is not achieved by filling it with food that has been processed beyond recognition. Wholesome ingredients for all the senses are vitally important in our life. Just as important as taking care of these physical needs, we also need to be fully present in our life, and to realize our highest potential: we need to address our inner self. Finding our connection to the divine source and cherishing our soul is one side of the coin. As we master this side we raise our awareness. On the other side of the coin are our physical and emotional limitations that call out for a therapy that addresses our healing on a similarly holistic level. That is where homeopathy comes in. Homeopathy can answer our most profound questions about our health and well-being. Awareness is not necessarily enough to remove energetic debris from our body. Homeopathy is capable of addressing the energetic core on the innermost level and can gently begin to reorganize unbalanced energies on the mental, emotional, and physical levels. As we become aware and address what's happening on all these levels, we may shine with the glowing light of utmost clarity and consciousness.

THE CHALLENGE

One of the challenges that faces homeopathy is that it does not fit the mold of the worldview we have been accustomed to. Understanding the workings of homeopathy requires a paradigm shift from the old and well-known path. Dr. Timothy Dooley's introductory book on homeopathy, *Flat Earth Medicine,* uses the metaphor of sailors who were trained to think the earth was flat and that if they sailed the globe they would fall off the edge into nothingness. Imagine the courage needed to go on that first voyage and take the risk of that jump! It took a visionary mind to be the captain of the ship, but finding a willing crew must have been a challenging undertaking. The book *Presence* addresses this issue in more modern terms. The authors are consultants to large corporations and global organizations, and they help them maneuver into sustainable directions. They write:

> *Most change initiatives that end up going nowhere don't fail because they lack grand visions and noble intentions. They fail because people can't see the reality they face. Likewise, studies of corporate mortality show that most Fortune 500 companies fail to outlast a few generations of management not because of resource constraints but because they are unable to "see" the threats they face and the imperative to change. "The signals of threat are always abundant and recognized by many" says Arie de Geus. "Yet somehow they fail to penetrate the corporate immune system response to reject the unfamiliar.*[1]

Just as corporations are unable to see the threats they face in business, people are unable to see the threats in their health. The state of health in modern man is alarming, but too few people are ready to look for any perspective other than the conventional way. "The signals of threat" are many, which we can see just by looking at the accelerating rate of chronic diseases in modern society. Still, most people still want to sail on the

---

[1] Senge, Peter, Scharmer, C. Otto, Jaworski, Joseph, Flowers, Betty Sue, *Presence, Exploring Profound Change in People, Organizations, and Society.* Cambridge, MA: SOL, (2004) p. 29.

"safe" waters of the flat earth; they are reluctant to take that jump into the abyss.

You have the opportunity today to chart a very different course. I invite you to explore homeopathy, even if it sounds unfamiliar to you at first. This book will provide you a compass. I invite you to try incorporating the ideas that form the backbone of homeopathy into your everyday health care. Then, see if you fall off the edge of the earth, or if you suddenly see something you never thought you would!

The System of Homeopathy

Vital Force

The resting point of our body is health. That is the state our vital force, the energy that enlivens our body, is moving us toward. Our body is the instrument through which we can achieve the ultimate goal of our existence. When our body is not in this ideal state, the vital force is working hard to return to it. When the vital force is struggling, symptoms appear in our body. These symptoms are the body's way of communicating to us that there is something not right. When there is no struggle, there are no symptoms. A gentle well-being reigns in our body: we feel at ease, healthy, like everything is in its right place.

Indeed it is. This state is the goal homeopathic treatment is working toward. In the chapters ahead, you will see glimpses of the state of well-being. You will find road maps showing you how to get there. The destination is the state of health. What are the signs that can help guide you to see the road? What are the subtle or not so subtle signs in an illness that can hint at the possible image of health? We are going to explore these signs through the examples of real people who choose to follow a homeopathic route to wellness.

THE ESSENCE

The focus of homeopathic understanding is to see what is unique in a person. That's different from the conventional approach, which constructs its road map by finding what is common in people. Adequate levels of measurements, daily allowances of certain nutrients and the most suitable medication for a certain disease are established. Once you suffer from an ailment, you are categorized by the ailment and its symptoms will be treated. The goal of conventional treatment is to free you from those symptoms and get your measurements back to the normal range.

Homeopathy views health differently. Instead of trying to match one with pre-labeled notions and disease categories it is aimed at addressing what is unique in that person. In this way it finds the unique essence in the midst of common features. Once that unique essence is addressed the body will go back to its natural resting place: health. Symptoms will disappear not because they were counteracted but because the whole organism came to a healthy, balanced state where the vital force does not need to work hard to get back there; it does not need to create the symptoms anymore.

As we explore case studies of actual people, we will learn how to find the unique core individuality in each situation. At the same time we will also explore how this individuality shows up everywhere in the same person. Each symptom carries something common, which is characteristic of all other symptoms of the person. This common element is the key to the health of the whole organism. By studying the person's individuality in depth, we come to see the wholeness of the individual.

HOMEOPATHY – CURING WITH SIMILARS

Homeopathy is a system of healing that is capable of restoring health in a gentle way. It has been practiced for over 200 years. Going back even further, we find that the same principles that are the cornerstones of the science of homeopathy were used – consciously or unconsciously – for thousands of years. Homeopathy means "similar suffering." The core idea is that healing agents are present in the universe and the healer's task is to find the matching pair: what heals what. If one lacks health there is a substance in nature that carries the corresponding healing energy for that particular state of dis-ease. This substance carries similar energetic qualities as the diseased state of the person and is therefore capable of bringing the sick back to health through its similarity rather than counter-action.

This idea is similar to the energetic undercurrents in martial arts. The winning technique in the fight is achieved through understanding the opponent's energy and flowing with it to bring the opponent to defeat. Opposing by force, in contrast, takes more energy from us and can be damaging not only to the opponent but to ourselves as well.

In physics, waves behave in a similar fashion. Ripples caused by a pebble dropped in water can be neutralized by creating waves in sync with the original waves. Creating counteracting waves may cause an impressive splash but it will take longer for the water surface to calm down again and reach its original resting state.

DISEASE

Homeopaths interpret the word disease literally as "lack of ease." We are looking for the difference between the diseased state and the healthy – what makes the diseased condition different from the ideal, healthy state of a person? We search for the core imbalance that manifests in mental, emotional and physical symptoms. The goal is to eliminate the imbalance rather than fight the manifestations: the symptoms. A sick person is mainly troubled by these symptoms and would like to get rid of them, but if our sole focus is on the symptoms we lose sight of the big picture. Because the surfacing symptoms are governed by the core imbalance, eliminating it will stop the appearance of those symptoms. The big picture includes the core as well as its manifestations. When we keep that picture in sight, we will find the governing core and we will make sure that we follow through until all the symptoms fade away.

HEALING

As I mentioned at the start of the chapter, the vital force is working in all of us to maintain the flow of health. If we are at ill health the vital force is working to bring us back to good health. Homeopathic treatment is guided by the same purpose, by providing a helping hand to the vital force. Homeopathic remedies gently work to bring the body back to healthy balance. Remedies are given in minute doses – just enough to give that extra little nudge the vital force needs to bring the organism back to health. Homeopathic remedies do their job in a truly gentle way. They do not introduce a new force into the system that knocks out the disease-causing agents. They affect the natural self-healing mechanism, giving it an extra boost. That is how homeopathic treatment follows the natural direction the body is taking.

Instead of trying to block the wind from causing harm to our livelihood we can build windmills and use the energy of the wind to achieve constructive goals. This same principle is true in all areas of life. Opposing something costs us energy, while going with it and gently guiding it in a positive direction creates energy. Keep this fundamental principle in mind while reading this book. Healing with homeopathy is based on the genuine flow of nature. When we follow it, we can comprehend the remarkable complexity of life's simplicity.

THE EMERGENCE OF THE
SENSATION METHOD

SENSATION

The master plan that creates the guiding force in homeopathic healing is what we call the *vital sensation*. When homeopaths listen to their clients' words describing their dis-ease, they are listening to words that describe the inner sensation. The inner sensation is something that you experience throughout your physical, emotional, mental and spiritual reality. This is the core sensation through which you filter the world around you. It's how you perceive good, bad, pleasant, painful, exciting and boring, fear and joy, your body and your spirit, your neighbors and your pets, your dreams and your job, competition and performance, smells and sights and other life circumstances. Reality is something you perceive; it is not a fixed experience for all. Reality changes according to the filter you look through at it. This filter is the core sensation, the vital sensation. Otto Scharmer, a leading expert on organizational learning, calls the same phenomena the "blind spot" in his book *Theory U*. Talking about leaders he worked with he explains:

...what counts is not only what leaders do and how they do it but their 'interior condition,' the inner place from which they operate or the source from which all their actions originate. (...) if we were to ask the question "From what source does our action come?" most of us would be unable to provide an answer. We can't see the source from which we operate; we aren't aware of the place from which our attention and intention originate.[2]

This *source* is what the homeopath has to find in each person. This vital sensation holds the key to the homeopathic remedy

---

[2] Scharmer, C. Otto, *Theory U, Leading from the Future as It Emerges.* Cambridge, MA: Sol (2007) p. 7.

that is capable of cleaning that filter, consequently bringing relief. Ease and health, the person's natural state, will prevail.

Healing through homeopathy aims to dissolve the central disturbance, the deep-seated imbalance blocking the healthy state. The homeopathic remedy addresses this core imbalance. Once it is corrected, the body can return to its natural state of being. The time needed will vary from person to person depending on the general well-being of the organism. The remedy induces this process and the rest is the workings of the body's own self-healing mechanism. It's important to understand that the remedy is not aimed at chasing after each problem and trying to solve them one by one. Rather, homeopaths believe that everything that ails a person can be traced back to the energetic core. Once that is returned, the body will heal itself – on the mental, emotional and physical levels. The vital sensation helps the homeopath to find the remedy capable of initiating that healing process, the individual path that person needs to take to be healed.

THE PROCESS

The process that a homeopath follows to elicit the core sensation is to find a substance in nature that has a similar energy to it. Homeopaths have been working on understanding the energetic blueprints of substances in nature since homeopathy was founded two hundred years ago. Samuel Hahnemann, the founder of homeopathy, realized that symptoms created by a crude substance could be healed if the same substance was administered in minutely diluted homeopathic doses. These doses are called remedies. Each remedy can potentially heal thousands of symptoms, given that they arise from a common vital sensation. After thorough study of the remedies and the corresponding symptoms, the names of the remedies were collected and catalogued in the Homeopathic Materia Medica. By studying the symptoms of a remedy, we get a glimpse into the energetic world of the substances that remedies come from. The Homeopathic Materia Medica is a gigantic database of symptoms. Homeopaths sought a simpler way to sort through it. As a result, many great thinkers in homeopathy grouped the remedies according to certain rules.

The first attempt to group remedies was made by Hahnemann, who introduced the notion of miasms. He found that people that had some common traits in their personality and physical makeup shared some similarities with their ancestors' disease histories. Based on this finding, he named these traits by the names of those diseases. This idea was subsequently expanded, and we will discuss it later in this chapter.

Another approach is to group remedies by the natural category of the original substance, such as remedies coming from spiders, snakes, metals, acids, etc. Some categories are broader and are based on some quality of the original substance, which does not necessarily come from the same natural order. An example is the "drug remedies." Remedies made from coffee, chocolate, alcohol and the plant sources of poppy or cannabis belong to this group.

Location of the original substance is another way to see similarities between remedies. For example, sea remedies come from mineral, animal and plant sources that share the ocean as their home.

Remedies also are grouped by the part of the population they are most commonly used for, such as remedies for hormonal imbalances in women, remedies for behavior problems in children, etc. A useful grouping for the novice is according to the acute ills that most often bring about states that correspond to the remedy, such as headache remedies, teething remedies or remedies for coughs, injuries, burns, bladder infections, poison ivy, etc.

As homeopathy gained more popularity in the 1800s, and people used it for long-term health care management, some polychrests emerged. Polychrests are the most often used remedies that homeopaths describe as general personality archetypes. These remedies have wide spread use, they cover many aspects of the human body including a broad spectrum of emotional, physical, and mental symptoms. They usually have a fully built personality profile and affect the whole organism as opposed to remedies that are used in specific situations and used less frequently than polychrests. James Tyler Kent, an American homeopath of the era, was one of the first to work extensively on describing all aspects of these polychrests.

DOCTRINE OF SIGNATURES AND OTHER APPROACHES

One aspect of healing with similars is the realization that there is a connection between the energy of a substance and the energy of the person in need of healing. Remedies carry the energetic blueprint of their original substance. We can classify them in a similar fashion to how they are classified in their original form, the substance in nature. The idea of classifying remedies according to their sources is not new. Some authors have called it the "doctrine of signatures" and it has been utilized by several homeopaths extensively. Misha Norland, a contemporary British homeopath, approaches remedies this way. In this approach the emphasis is not only on the symptoms a remedy can heal but also on broadening the understanding of these remedies by studying their natural habitat, qualities, behaviors. We can draw parallels with the personality of the people who benefit from the remedy.

Italian homeopath Massimo Mangialavori groups remedies according to their common characteristics regardless of their natural habitat. For example, in the group of sea remedies he includes other minerals in the grouping if they share basic characteristics. Or, based on the same idea, he adds some remedies made of salts of zinc to the snake group.

Some would name the similarity between the physical characteristics of a plant and the physical manifestations in the person. For example, a person who needs a plant with yellow flowers manifests with a condition with yellow bile and jaundice. American homeopath Paul Herscu has worked out a system called "cycles and segments." This system works mainly with the first approach we discussed, when the homeopath focuses on the grouping of symptoms rather than their similarities to the source. Herscu filters through the symptoms according to the essence they are manifesting. If there was a discharge in a certain body part or excessive restlessness, even though one is a physical manifestation and the other is an emotional restlessness, they belong to the same segment because they are the same phenomena expressed as different symptoms. They both express discharge.

All these approaches have helped the practice of homeopathy and its practitioners to better utilize the Materia Medica. Once a practitioner masters one or more approach, they can be extremely useful tools in prescribing. Nevertheless, the most groundbreaking classification in the history of homeopathy has come with Rajan Sankaran's system of classifying the remedies according to the kingdoms in which their crude substances are found. The difference between the way the doctrine of signatures was used before this method and working with the Sensation Method is that we identify the kingdom on the sensation level. It means that we do not look for superficial similarities between the source and the person. Rather, we elicit the sensation they experience reality with and match that with the characteristics of the source. This is an important distinction. If this matching did not occur at this level we could pick any random element in a person and match it with a remedy. Some practitioners who have heard about this method and try to practice it without understanding this important distinction have made some embarrassing mistakes. To understand this distinction, one has to be familiar with the seven levels of experience.

LEVELS OF EXPERIENCE

The key to the Sensation Method lies in the structure of the initial interview. When we conduct a homeopathic interview we take the client by the hand and walk them through their inner reality step by step, guiding them deeper into the levels of experience. The first level people usually start telling their story at is by naming their ailment. The next step is when they describe the symptoms in detail: conditions, how their ailment appears or improves, the location, the severity of those and other descriptions. One level deeper, people talk about feelings – the emotions these symptoms evoke or are born into. At this level people tend to take a broader route and relate their experience in more general terms from the emotional perspective. Most people have strong emotional reactions and are quite aware of them, so this is a level of experience people can talk freely about. One step beyond this is the level of images – the situations the person relates to. This is the first level that we do not tend to go to easily in casual conversation. It can be a stretch for many people to realize that underneath our emotional reactions there are fixed images that we unconsciously believe in. This is the layer people draw from when describing their situation in metaphors.

Once this level is well described, we go further into the realm of sensations. At this level people relate to the physical sensation a certain image, dream or situation brings forth. This level correlates to the local sensations and brings out the global sensation that manifests everywhere in the person. Without reaching this level we cannot be sure of the core sensation that feeds the images, the emotions, the symptoms and the ailment the person is suffering from. On this level, then, we can identify the kingdom with precision. Let's take a look at how we classify our remedies on this level.

THE BASICS OF THE KINGDOMS

The scientific mind of man has created categories in order to classify nature. These categories are called kingdoms. There are three main categories: the mineral kingdom, the plant kingdom and the animal kingdom. Since homeopathic remedies come from sources of nature, this classification fits our remedies as well. The three categories carry qualities that are based on the natural order of kingdoms. Our remedies carry the resemblance to their crude sources, so our categories are also based on, but not bound only to, the qualities of substance. Humanity perceives life in material terms, whereas we know that all around and within us is energy. Our perception is what creates substance, thereby enabling us to see, feel, touch or smell these substances. Even though we are not always aware of the basic nature of these substances, the energy is nevertheless there. In homeopathy we deal with these energies. We use the language of our material world as tools to describe what we feel and what we heal, but it is not on this level that healing actually takes place.

Eckhart Tolle, a spiritual teacher and author of the best-selling book *The Power of Now,* describes an energetic manifestation of humans in the most elegant way. He coined the term "pain body," meaning the ego and mind that we identify our whole being with. When we identify ourselves with this part of ourselves, we create a habit based on emotionally charged reaction from which we cannot break free. The further our path takes us in identifying with this pain body, the harder it is to cut ourselves off from it. But if we choose to, we can let it go.[3]

Curiously, this pain body is a very similar manifestation to what Rajan Sankaran calls the "Other Song" in humans. It is also referred to as the ego. These are terms that describe a part of ourselves that takes over our whole being, our consciousness. It is a challenging force that we often fail to recognize and thus we give up our true self – our soul – and as we become influenced by this force we get out of balance. Once we are out of balance, the path to dis-ease is open and we tend to fall ill on some level. Sooner or later our whole being will be affected by the imbalance, making it difficult for us to see our way back to the healthy state, the balanced state, the state without ego. The state we are meant to be in.

---

[3] Tolle, Eckhart, *The Power of Now, A Guide to Spiritual Enlightenment.* Vancouver: Namaste Publishing (1999) pp. 36–41.

The attempt to identify this force in homeopathy is eliciting the energy, the resonance that created the core imbalance. That is the *Other Song*, the blueprint of a homeopathic remedy. *Other Song* is a telling name because we hear the words of a person describing something different than a healthy human state. In health, a human being experiences reality without restrictions, without fears and concerns; all the organs of the body work in harmony and we do not need to pay attention to their workings. This is the ideal state. In homeopathy we do not draw a line between manifestations on the physical, mental or emotional levels. Once the balance is broken, the same underlying disturbance manifests at different locations, thus creating symptoms on all these levels. You will see in the illustrating examples that the same energy can be seen in a physical complaint and in an emotional or mental phenomenon.

Let's look at how Tolle describes the phenomenon of breaking free from the pain body. His description is an illustration of how energies can get healed, and it's very similar to homeopathic thinking about cure.

It is your conscious Presence that breaks the identification with the pain-body. When you don't identify with it, the pain-body can no longer control your thinking and so cannot renew itself anymore by feeding on your thoughts. The pain-body in most cases does not dissolve immediately, but once you have severed the link between it and your thinking, the pain-body begins to lose energy. (…) The energy that was trapped in the pain-body then changes vibrational frequency and is transmuted into Presence. (…) Regardless of what you say or do or what face you show to the world, your mental-emotional state cannot be concealed. Every human being emanates an energy field that corresponds to his or her inner state…[4]

That energy that was trapped inside the pain body is what we homeopaths call a "remedy state." It is that other song that is playing along with the human song within. It is the unnecessary

---

[4] Tolle, Eckhart, *A New Earth: Awakening to Your Life's Purpose.* Vancouver: Namaste Publishing (2005) p. 161.

inner vibration that is the core problem and that needs to be eliminated in order to have a clear, healthy vibrational state. Sometimes a good homeopathic interview can "sever the link" Tolle is talking about. The person reaches the sensation level, the level at which they can identify that sensation that resides in the core and does not let them be free and healthy. Usually, however, this short-term severing resulting from the interviewing process is not enough. The remedy provides the right amount of energy in the right frequency that can remove this connection permanently. Sometimes, when the person is chronically ill, the sensation gets overwhelming and the "other song" occupies more than the healthy part of the person. As Tolle puts it, "in illness the energy is low and the ego can strive (…) in chronic illness some people never recover from identifying with the ego – it becomes a permanent part of their false self."[5]

In this situation, when the person's energy is far beyond the possibility of restoring all-encompassing health, a remedy might not be able to remove that imbalance anymore. This happens in cases that are deemed to be incurable. Homeopathic remedies might be able to bring relief and alleviate the symptoms and create more well-being in the person, but total cure is much less likely.

In the following chapters we will discuss in more detail the various expressions of the subtle underlying energy. You will read about the kingdoms as they refer to human behaviors and sensations in health and disease. This classification corresponds to the diverse survival techniques species have developed. What makes a mineral a mineral or a plant a plant? What makes animals different from other kingdoms? The answer is in the specific way these creatures cope with survival.

---

[5] Tolle, Eckhart, *A New Earth*. p. 124.

THE MINERAL KINGDOM

People who need mineral remedies see reality as structure and view themselves lacking something in their structure. Their function depends on their structure. Their sheer existence, identity, security, role in society, performance and responsibilities are perceived in different levels of structure. They feel as though they are missing something to be perfectly well, to perform or carry responsibility for themselves and others. They might feel they had it all figured out but are losing it now. These are all variations on the same theme: do I have what it takes? Even if they feel secure they are concerned with issues of this realm: their inner ability to withstand the pressure of life. Minerals in nature are qualified by their ability to withstand pressure and may be formed as gases, metals or other non-metals. Their structure is what defines their existence.

THE PLANT KINGDOM

Survival of plants depends on their ability to sense what is happening in their environment. They are growing in one place and have to adapt to conditions of moisture, such as extreme flooding or dryness, strong winds and fluctuations in temperature – from the heat of the blazing sun to the freezing cold. Their survival depends on their ability to react to those influences around them. People who need plant remedies are sensitive to their environment and tend to be reactive. When they talk, they emphasize their inner sensations as reactions to the outside influence. Naturally, in working with people we often see reactions to other people, but we also see physical sensitivity to temperature and noise, as well as pollens and other elements of nature. People who need remedies from the plant kingdom do not talk about their inner ability to withstand pressure as minerals do. They describe how outside forces affect them.

THE ANIMAL KINGDOM

The animal kingdom is based on the food chain, or survival of the fittest: the stronger wins, the weaker looses. But who is the victim and who is the aggressor? In most cases it is two sides of the same coin. Within one individual there is a sense of being weaker than someone else and in other instances they are the stronger party. In cases of animal remedies, people even experience their physical ailments as an entity that is going to win or lose against them. You know the expression: "This headache is killing me." This could be uttered by anybody but once someone uses expressions like this frequently, a homeopath can use it as the key to the door that opens to a person's inner world.

Animals, and people who need animal remedies, deal with territory and survival. They often remark on another person's appearance and dress with the purpose of seduction or seeking attention. If they are concerned with their position in society, it is not about their inner structure (as in a mineral remedy) but rather a competition for power over others.

SUBKINGDOMS

Based on the specific means of survival, we classify remedies into subgroups within the kingdoms. This is done by the same subcategories that the sciences of biology and chemistry use: in minerals we use the lines and columns of the periodic table; in plants we use the plant families; and in animals we use the classes like mammals, birds, reptiles, insects, etc. Just as qualities of the kingdoms correspond to qualities of human behavior, these more specific qualities of the subkingdoms will manifest through the remedy's picture.

Miasms

The next cornerstone of the Sensation Method is the classification by miasms. Miasms are the coping mechanisms a person tends to use in approaching his or her problems and obstacles. As homeopaths, it is not enough to determine the sensation in the complaint. We also have to identify the degree, the depth and the severity of it. People with similar sensations will cope with their problems in varying ways. This coping mechanism is what we call a miasm. We will learn more about miasms when we discuss the Plants cases, describing how the specific remedy was picked for the person being treated.

The Techniques of a Homeopath

Words

The primary tools of homeopathy are words. Other healing modalities use other tools: manipulating energy channels or pressure points in the body, using pressure of fingers and hands or needle points, visual art or music in art therapies, movement and other aspects of the physical body in bodywork. In homeopathy we talk. We ask questions and listen to what the person has to say. And more than just listening to *what* they say, we listen to *how* they say it. To elicit important qualities we need to listen to the words the person is using. There is a certain aspect of words we use that draws us to them. If we listen to the words we frequently use, we begin to hear some recurrent themes and so might understand more about ourselves than with emotional exploration. Sometimes emotions can send us on winding roads of our spirit, and we might get lost. A shortcut can be found when we listen to the simple utterances we use in telling our complicated story. That's what homeopaths do.

In homeopathic case-taking, we ask patients to tell us about their inner sensation. When talking about their inner sensation, people can talk about it without the pain attached to it. It just is. They can talk about it without getting emotionally involved in it. They talk about it from outside that pain-body Eckhart Tolle (1999) talked about. Helping a person talk in this manner is an important attribute of homeopathic case-taking. By going into the sensation without the emotions attached to it, we can explore it without so much drama. The process goes deep, exact and does not cause suffering. Once the sensation is identified, it can be addressed. This might explain how some people get well after the interview, even if they have not yet received their remedy. Usually, however, this effect of the interview is short-lived; long-term benefits are experienced only after taking the appropriate homeopathic remedy.

Hand Gestures

Another great tool that shows underlying energy is following the hand gestures a person uses. Body movements are manifesting the same energy as words, in a slightly different format. When we use our hands while explaining something or putting more emphasis on our thoughts and words, we unknowingly use a telling venue of energy. Energetic patterns that express our inner sensations are manifesting not only through words we use or ailments we suffer from. The body is embedded in these energies, and all our movements are governed by them. That is why often, when people are not sure how to express a feeling they first gesture with their hands and then the expression in words follows it. Most often these patterns are unconscious, which is exactly why they help us opening a door to the innermost sensations that we are not aware of but which affect our whole being.

Doodling

Doodling is one of the tools used for confirming the vital sensation or creating the right state of mind to talk about the vital sensation. A doodle is an abstract drawing that the person creates absentmindedly while in the presence of the homeopath. Usually, we tend to doodle when we're bored or while our mind is wandering without consciously thinking of the drawing. Since a doodle is not planned or conscious, and is in a way *nonsense*, it exactly matches the kind of experience we are looking for in our homeopathic case-taking. Using these doodles we can reach the vital sensation. This can be done at the beginning or the end of the interview, as an encouragement to enter the state of the sensations or as a confirmation to see whether the person arrives at the same sensation through the doodle as through telling their story.

In this approach, the client doodles something with a black pen on a white piece of paper. If he or she has a recurrent scheme of doodles they should doodle that. They can draw several doodles and then pick one that has the most impact on them. The next step is for the person to just look at the doodle without thinking or interpreting it. It is an intimate time when only the person and the doodle are present, so to speak, and the person is asked to concentrate on the experience, the sensation the doodle brings out. After this the client is asked to explain their experience. If they talk about the same experience they described earlier, and they use gestures as well, we know we are in the right track. Otherwise, we can use this experience as a starting point for further discussion.

Drawing a doodle can have a healing effect on its own because when a person looks at it, they experience their own sensation as in a meditative state. Homeopaths often observe that after drawing the doodle the person revitalizes or feels better, as they experienced something profound in their inner world.

The tone of voice we use, the way we dress and the way we move are all expressions of the energy we carry within. When homeopaths listen to the words one speaks, and apply all these other tools to deepen their understanding, they will get a clearer picture of that inner essence they are looking for.

CASE-TAKING

Case-taking is the first step in understanding a person's inner reality. The flow of the interview is set by the patient during the interview, with occasional guiding questions or requests for more specific information. The homeopath usually lets the patient lead the way in this process, instead of trying to fit them into a preset mold. The homeopath wants to find out about the inner experience of the person regarding the chief complaint. Once that is covered the flow of the interview proceeds to whatever areas the person takes it to. As you will see in the cases discussed in detail, there are several complaints and areas one talks about. The inner sensation – the core – can be reached from anywhere. In fact, the goal of case-taking is to reach the same spot from all manifesting areas. If a person has arthritis, depression, recurrent colds and some inability to concentrate, describing these problems one by one will point to the same vital sensation. Underneath each of our individual problems is the same vital sensation.

Once that vital sensation is elicited, the remedy will address that sensation. Consequently, once the healing response starts, that sensation will dissolve and bring healing to the manifesting ailments. All this will not emerge when talking to a person casually. Deep probing is required in order to elicit symptoms on this level.

SOURCE LANGUAGE

Reaching a level where the person thinks their story does not make sense anymore is a very important aspect of the Sensation Method. We have to arrive at a point during the interview when there is enough trust and rapport between homeopath and client for this to happen. It is important to have this comfort zone; otherwise, the person telling their story would feel uncomfortable and leave the level of nonsense, escaping back to "'reality,'" to the world of common sensibility. But on the level of common sense many people tell very similar stories, thus losing the individuality we need to comprehend in a person in order to arrive at a single remedy that is able to heal their unique, individual imbalances. In fact, this "nonsense" makes a lot of sense out of the human context. That is exactly why it demonstrates so well the connection between the person and the source of the remedy they need. They are talking about the attributes of the source of that remedy.

This is what we call source language. Decoding this level is an art the homeopath needs to be skilled at. There are rules by which it is possible to differentiate between plants in the mountains that a person may enjoy looking at or, if they describe a plant source, which is the remedy they need. Many people like animals and could describe their nature, habitat and behaviors, but they do not need an animal remedy. On the other hand, some people do need a remedy made of that animal source and they describe their inner sensations according to the nature, habitat and behaviors of that animal. This is a fine art of distinction that the homeopath needs to develop.

FLOW OF INTERVIEW

There is no fixed pattern of case-taking, no set questions we need to ask our clients. Nevertheless, we want to touch upon all the Levels of Experience as discussed earlier. There is a natural flow that takes people through their story. In the beginning of the interview we ask about the nature of the complaint. Once that is described, we further question specific aspects of it. Nowadays, health care consumers are very well informed. With the widespread use of the Internet, information is just a click away. Consequently, people tend to know a great deal about their condition. However, this does not replace the actual symptoms one experiences. These symptoms are more personal than the average, general description of an illness. People can go into minute details about their pains and discomforts. This is important terrain for the homeopath, who can then dive deeper into even more personal experience of these symptoms. This is the starting points from which people then usually describe their emotional circumstances of their complaints. Once they are talking about the emotions it is just one step further to understand their beliefs that those emotions are based on.

This is a depth which typical conversation seldom reaches. It's the level at which we need to encourage our patients to go ahead and describe their inner reality, however absurd or unreasonable it might sound. For some, it is as senseless as dreams. It has vague relation to reality but they are not sure what the connection is. They do not act as predictably as they usually do in their waking life. Indeed, at this level people talk about their dreams, pictures, images of their daydreams, the goals they want to achieve, hobbies they enjoy, favorite movies, books, stories and heroes. Once a person is talking about these things they experience certain sensations. There is a reason we feel good at the sight of an awe-inspiring piece of art or scenery. There is a reason we engage in a particular sport or activity. Once we can tackle that sensation the activity brings up, we are in a very different realm than describing symptoms of a disease. In this realm we can navigate through with ease; there are no norms we have to comply with. At this level it is also easy to name the sensation and the opposite of it, which brings on unpleasant associations. Often two polarities can be elicited here, and that can secure our understanding of the vital sensation. We arrive at the root of the problem, the key to healing.

A REMINDER

This book explores the healing potential of homeopathy; it presents success that homeopathic treatment can achieve. It is important to emphasize that while the cases portrayed in this book yielded good result: the clients benefited from homeopathic treatment, and made significant changes in their lives and well-being, it is not always the case. Sometimes the key to solving the case eludes the practitioner and healing does not happen easily and quickly. In some instances healing crises happen, which makes the journey towards health harder or less comfortable. Adverse reactions happen in any healing modality, and homeopathy is not an exception. Homeopathy is well-known for its gentle healing and infrequent adverse reactions but it does not mean that these never happen. Comprehensive knowledge of the system of homeopathy and mindful practice are the keys to successful treatment outcomes.

CHAPTER 2
A DEEPER UNDERSTANDING OF THE MINERAL KINGDOM

In this chapter we will look at three illustrative cases where the person needed a mineral remedy. We will see how and why mineral remedies are fascinating examples of how the natural order of minerals translates into our homeopathic understanding of personality types of people.

Minerals are elements or combinations of elements. All the elements are organized in the periodic table, which is divided into rows and columns. The elements are placed in order of their atomic weight: the ones in the top row are the lightest and toward the bottom of the periodic table they are getting heavier and heavier. One could say the further we go down in the periodic table, the people who need those remedies will have more and more "weight." We're not referring to body weight but rather that they will carry more weight on their shoulders in terms of responsibility, or the ability to care for themselves and others. The pressure they feel they are dealing with in their everyday life increases as well.

In our homeopathic understanding, we draw a parallel between stages of human development and the rows in the periodic table. The elements of the first row deal with existence. People who need one of these remedies describe their ailments as elemental questions of being. They feel that their existence is so questionable they feel lonely, abandoned or unrecognized. The second row of elements mainly deals with issues of detachment from the source. These are expressed as the need or inability of moving apart from another entity, often a person's mother or family. The third row deals with the developmental stage of identity: as a person matures they establish an identity for themselves in society. The next step, the fourth row, works toward creating security for themselves and, once that is achieved for others, for their loved ones. Issues with financial security and safety come up in these remedies. The fifth-row remedies have all the previous preliminaries down, so they crave adventure. These people are creators of the new and beautiful: artists, speakers, actors and researchers. The sixth row has all the above under control. They hold great responsibility. Heads of organizations, bankers, leaders and politicians are a few examples that might be typically included in this category. When talking about their physical complaints, these people will describe their ailments in similar terms to their general view on reality.

Each mineral is found at a crossing point of a row and a column. Within a row there is a natural increase, peak and decline in success. The issue is established by the theme of the row and the specific remedy is pinpointed by the level of their success according to the column. So, when a person is talking to me, I have to decide what kingdom the person's remedy is in. It is as if the story they are telling me goes through a filter. When I hear words that describe structure, my mind is ready to build a mineral picture. The art of this work is staying in that dangling moment of being ready for a mineral picture to emerge while at the same time staying open to the other kingdoms. The more words coming in that confirm the mineral kingdom, the more ready I am to act on the basis of those words. And the more words I hear in general, the more aware I become of the structure they are talking about. I start understanding what the lack is that they perceive in their reality. Where they perceive that their structure is standing, where are the flaws of it? Where is it collapsing or breaking? How much pressure is it placed under? I keep asking questions so the person will specifically tell me the inner sensation in all their symptoms, and eventually they arrive at the sensation that cannot be further described with new dimensions. Further inquiry will only yield more of the same depth, the same qualities, the same sensation.

Once it becomes clear where in the process of human development this person is struggling – the point they cannot pass without help – we know we are at the right spot in the periodic table.

There is another aspect of the way a person talks in this process. They often speak in a unique language that actually describes the original substance from which the remedy was made. People talking this way experience reality in a way that can be related to that original substance. They will often talk about relationships, the need to give something or be attached to somebody. Curiously the image of atoms and electrons comes to mind. A person who needs a remedy like magnesium or sodium needs to connect to someone, just as the sodium and magnesium ions need to pick up an electron on their outer shell because they lack one. A person who needs the remedy Natrum muriaticum, which originates from common salt (chloride of sodium), has issues on one hand with needing another person to feel their own identity because they believe they cannot exist without that person. On the other hand, they also feel betrayed by that person. This makes them close up and experience waves of emotions within, not letting the flood of tears show on the surface. Natrum muriaticum is a classical remedy for grief. The central feeling in this remedy is that one has a sense of being betrayed by the people they love and depend on. If you look at the periodic table of elements (at the end of the book) you will see that the two components, sodium and chlorine are found at two opposite ends of the table. The difference in qualities of the elements explains the dual nature of this remedy. One has a lack, the other has excess. These two opposites build up the Natrum muriaticum picture.

Following are three actual cases related to choosing remedies from the mineral kingdom. These people came to see me with different complaints and received remedies made from different minerals. In all cases, however, the way they describe their complaints is characteristic of the mineral kingdom. Only their individual situations differ. One is from the end of the second line, the second is from the beginning of the fifth line, and the third case if from the beginning of the sixth line.

IN NEED OF OXYGEN

The issues for the remedies of the first two rows symbolize the stages of conception and birth. A sense of identity has not yet developed at these stages so it is not easy to comprehend the essence of these remedies as structure. Structure, along with identity, develops after separation from the mother. What we see in the complaints of these people – in symbolic terms – is the lack of the structure and the need for it.

The first line of the periodic table consists of two elements: Hydrogen and Helium. The essential question for people who need one of these remedies relates to their existence. All their issues boil down to the most basic questions: To be or not to be? Am I or am I not? Do I exist or don't I exist? The answer comes as we step into the second line of the periodic table and we remedies that have established their presence, their existence. Their goal is the next phase in development: detaching from the source. In symbolic terms they need to separate from the mother figure. As we go along this line, the separation unfolds: the first element, Lithium, cannot detach from the source. In all their doings in life they need someone who stands there for them and helps them through life by solving their problems. They feel safe and protected and do not intend to leave this safe heaven. As we proceed along the line, Beryllium, the next remedy, knows that detachment is inevitable but extremely scared of it. In Boron, Carbon, Nitrogen and Oxygen, this separation continues. Fluorine and Neon are fully separated from the source.

As we look at cases of these remedies we see physical complaints that have been resolved by using these images. Skin diseases that are viewed by the person as the inability to detach this layer or painful menstruation can be examples of this physical phenomenon. While most of the time these themes emerge as symbolic parallels to the birth process, it is important to realize that these remedies can be helpful in actual labor as well. For example, Carbo vegetabilis, a carbon remedy, is often used in infants and mothers with troublesome births. Let's look at the symbolic values of these themes.

The following example is the case of Fanny, a young woman who needed the remedy Oxygen. As you read her story listen beyond her words. If you train your mind to think the way homeopaths do, you will be able to distinguish two underlying stories: her life story as she would tell it to you in a casual conversation while chatting over coffee; and the underlying story, the one about separation from the source. Hear her words describing how she imagines her safe heaven as a bubble around her and how scary it is for her to leave that bubble. In symbolic terms this bubble is like the mother's womb. The images she shares describe her inner state. These are the images that her emotions and reactions stem from. This level of description is more telling than any complex explanation of her emotional realm. Her images also are accompanied by hand gestures, showing that these are important vehicles of communication for her; they truly come from her inner world. Notice that if you concentrate on this level of her story you will see the same pattern unfold on the mental, emotional and physical levels.

All the names in this book are fictional, and personal information has been altered to protect the clients' privacy. The interviews are concise versions of the original to enhance clarity.

Fanny is open to homeopathy; she is in tune with her feelings and understands the value of physical symptoms in the totality of the person. We build good rapport right in the beginning of her first visit.

– *How can I help you?*

– My fantasy is that you could help me quit smoking. I have been smoking since I was thirteen. There have been ups and downs but I could never quit. I cannot go without it. Smoking is the only unhealthy thing I do. Everybody hates it around me. But it is my best friend!

– *Tell me more about smoking. What does it mean for you?*

– I have done a lot of inner searching to find out what smoking meant for me. I think it is about giving myself space, giving myself oxygen. I feel I am not allowed to have space. And once I create space for myself I punish myself for having created it. I create it by doing healthy things: I do yoga, I push myself, I achieve things. But after that I have to have a cigarette. That is the punishment. I need to retract back to a level of comfort.

> Fanny makes a broad movement with her hand, pulling both arms towards her chest.

– *What do you mean by giving yourself oxygen?*
– I feel it is not okay to breathe. It is not okay to take space.
– *Not okay to take space?*
– As a metaphor, I think of my lungs. If I smoke that is a contradiction. I want to breathe; I want to take space. I will do it but then I will smoke. Smoking has to follow the activity through which I created space.
– *Tell me about creating space.*
– A lot of people in my family are not well; they have been stuck, not evolving. Here I am deciding not to live my life like that. That is my link to my family. They are a reminder for me. By distancing myself from them I am doing well. It is not perfect but it keeps me in balance.

> Her inner experience is that she can create herself as an individual if she rejects her family. She recreates herself as someone who needs her own space – she needs to breathe free; she needs oxygen. Strangely enough, she creates this space by smoking. This sounds like a contradiction. That is the reason I ask her about it. Once she explains that for her, smoking means creating safe space, where she can disconnect from her family members, we arrive at her inner world. It does not matter that smoking is not the most effective way of creating oxygen. The homeopath's job is to follow how she experiences her inner sensations. She does not want to be like her family.

They do not allow her to breathe. But she also recalls
that as soon as she manages to create her own space
and breathe some oxygen, she needs to retract back
to her familiar situation: her family.

– At this point in my life everything else is in place. At this point
smoking is just a physical addiction. One of my dreams is to
sing. Having a voice is a metaphor for being noticed in my family.
– *What do you mean by having a voice?*
– Saying how I feel. Setting a boundary.
– *Describe boundaries.*
– Saying no. Taking care of myself rather than saving the other
person. But I must say I feel guilty about it.
– *Say more about smoking.*
– Taking time for myself is pleasure. The cigarette symbolizes
that. When I smoke a cigarette I get a break; there are no
obligations. I have space. I have time off An image comes to my
mind: a bubble around me.

Here she again shows a round motion with her hands
drawing towards her chest.

– In that bubble I can be vulnerable. I can relax and be who I
am. It is calm. It feels like harmony. It is balanced.
– *Describe your experience in the bubble.*
– It is the sound of silence. Like in the mountains. Or when you
come to a building where the walls are very thick, so blocked.
Cannot hear anything. I can hear that silence. When you walk
into a building, there is that swallowed pressured air and it is
quiet.
– *What is the opposite of this?*
– Street sounds. People yelling. Metallic sounds. Machines.
– *How does that affect you?*
– It causes me stress. It is overload, too busy, too many details
that are not important.
– *How does it affect you?*
– It distracts me, resulting in me not being grounded in my body
and not breathing properly. It reminds me of my mother. She is

manic depressive: talks a lot, screams, breaks things. I want to get away from that. It is too over-stimulating. The city sounds remind me of that.

> The first image she uses in her story is the bubble. She puts an emphasis on this by showing the same gesture with her hands as when talking about retracting. She describes the sensations in that bubble as evoking the feelings in a womb, in contrast to the stimulus-full, noisy world into which a child is born. Inside the safe, quiet bubble she is calm, in harmony. Once she gets out from there, it is the mother's manic chatter, loud noises. That is too much for her. She yearns to be in the calm, quiet place. This is the place she is trying to get by creating space for herself.

– How do you feel when you are with your mother?
– There is no space for me. She comes to my skin; she has lots of needs. I cannot hear myself think or feel. It takes a lot of boundary-setting and pushing. I have to make that space. I should have this space naturally, but I have to work it all the time.

> We can almost see the protective womb around the fetus as opposed to this outside world that she now needs to deal with. She yearns for a bubble, a safe boundary around her. People come too close. She is not ready for them yet.

– Do you have the same feeling with other family members?
– With my sister I always have to protect myself, push away, be careful.

> As she says this, she uses the same hand gestures she used with the smoking creating space for her and the image of the building with thick walls. The two hand gestures are a protective circular motion, surrounding the inside and then the opening, the pushing out.

– With my father, I cannot allow myself to be vulnerable. I can't lean, can't rely on him. He is like rubber or seaweed. The most stressful aspect is that I cannot push. If I do, the "rubber" moves away. It is not going to be here.

— *How does it affect you?*

— It makes me angry, frustrated. As a child it made me rageful. I wanted him to respond — to hold and to contain my reaction. But he was not there to receive my anger. He was not there to hold that, to validate it. He denied that Mother was sick.

— *How did you feel about that?*

— I was angry. I needed a parent in order to know my own boundaries, to know my own self.

> This is what all the remedies in this line deal with: separating from the source and finding one's own boundaries. Now we have to locate the exact location in this process for Fanny. Her remedy will be at the point where she is stuck in this process. Imagine the birth process: she describes her urge to push at a firm surface, but it is not there. She is frustrated because there is nothing she can push at. On another level we can read her words saying that she needs a family and they are not there for her. She gets stuck at this stage because she does not get the healthy feedback from her family. She experiences it as they are not there. Thus she has to keep recreating this safe environment for herself, but she seems to fail in all her efforts.

— I could not explore my siblings. My mom was boundary-less, my father was like rubber. Rubber is the reflection of me. I could not learn interaction from either of them. I felt powerless. There was no hope. I was furious, very angry at the world. I wanted to know why everyone was crazy around me and the world did not seem to care. It was unfair. I wanted to look up to my parents but eventually I lost respect for them. My father lived in denial, he was not taking responsibility. I felt unprotected. A mountain could have exploded next to him and still he would not shift.

— *A mountain could have exploded next to him?*

— I felt like exploding! I felt full of rage, furious. But it seemed he had no feeling.

— How did that affect you?
— I was afraid that I was not going to be protected. I feel similarly with my son. His inability to accept my help is hurting me.
— Describe that feeling a little more.
— I am powerless. I am trying to help and he chooses not to accept the help. This way he is taking away my existence, who I am. It feels absurd. I cannot communicate with him and I cannot trust what happened.
— Say more about that.
— My general personality is to contain. I am a water sign in Astrology. I feel like I am a cup. I am very open to the world. And I fill, fill, fill, fill, until I overflow. Or I shut the cup and implode. I have carried my parents' baggage for a long time. My personality is to carry things. That contributed to my feeling of not being able to take space.

> The connection between these feelings will become clearer as we go on. On the surface it might seem that these references are unrelated, but for Fanny there is a common element that she is trying to convey. It is her sensation of pushing at something, relating to someone that does not have a firm consistency and thus moves out of the way when she pushes. This in turn creates a sense of not being protected. This is a quality of that water in the cup. It is a cupful of water only as long as the cup surrounds it. If there is no cup, there is no protection; there is no existence for the cupful of water (it will become a puddle).

— Tell more about not being able to take up space.
— I was a "good girl." I had a great, wild, free, safe childhood. We were catching frogs with my sister, lived in the wild.

> She uses the same gesture with the hands that she used when describing the bubble. This is her movement that expresses a safe environment. We know we are again at the same core sensation.

– Later my sister was diagnosed with schizophrenia. I lived through my childhood knowing something was wrong with her but nobody around me acknowledged it. At some point the happy childhood shifted and I turned into inhibition. It felt like I was a prisoner. It felt uncomfortable, not belonging.

> So the bubble is her safe place and her prison at the same time. She creates it to be safe but since it is a creation of the "pain body" (wounded energy body) it is not a true solution. It is a part of her remedy state, the imbalance she is found in. That is why both opposites are part of the problem and thus need to be addressed in the solution – the remedy she needs.

– When I was seven or nine my mom left for the U. S. I had a nightmare that she was crossing a street and got killed by a car. I was standing there and tried to catch her hand so I could help her to cross the street. When I woke up form this nightmare I called her in secret, so my father would not hear me. It was expensive to call. I just wanted to tell her that I wanted to take care of her. I was afraid for her. I felt her sadness, her misery.

> She was born and raised in Japan in an artist family. She was European but she did not belong to the diplomats or business people that came for a few years to live there. She lived there permanently, but she was not Japanese. To add to this, her parents came from two different cultures: one French and one American. She went from group to group, not belonging anywhere. Now it feels like the best gift in the world but back then she did not feel that way.

– I was an A student; everything was so easy. Then there was a shift at age nine. I was molested by a neighbor. It was a struggle, with a loss of ease in school. Then I also shifted with my sister. She made me worried. She would sneak out at night. My reaction was to become the good girl. I became too mature too early. I was introverted. I stopped taking risks. I gained a lot of weight and was ashamed of myself. At age thirteen I was obese. I was self-soothing by eating. I also think it had to do with taking up space. This was the time when I started smoking. I was forcing myself to smoke. I was choking and felt I could not master it! I was shut down a lot. I did not feel safe at home because there were always people. They were all extroverted, weird, odd people.

> The womb, the safe place, the home turns out to be not what it is supposed to be. So she looks for a substitute. She needs to create her own safe place.

– I always had some stable, generous people that shaped my life. I had millions of mothers. I felt good with my French neighbors. It was quiet in their house: safe and predictable.
– *Describe your need for safe, predictable space.*
– I needed it so I could go to my space, go to my dreams. So I could process and integrate. As an escape from my family I went to study in Paris. I was twenty years old, had no foundation, no ground beneath me. Interacting was too hurtful. I was an open wound in need to patch things up, to heal. I carried with me my parents' aversion to business. They were artists that did not understand anything about business. That is why I went to business school in Paris.

> Here again is the same theme of establishing her own identity by differentiating herself from her family. She needs to detach from the family in order to find herself. Regarding her physical complaints she recounts a few minor issues, like a chronic back injury, some seasonal allergies, psoriasis and retention of water. As a kid she had lots of ear infections and conjunctivitis. Then she describes the sensitivity of her skin.

– I can get tactile defensive. I don't want a person to touch me when I am angry. I need that space! I don't like if someone touches my skin.
– *What is the feeling?*
– It feels suffocating. I have had some curious dreams. My dad, sister and I were driving in a car on narrow roads, in the mountains, atop cliffs – very dangerous places. They were driving

but I was responsible. They were yelling at me. I was tied. My safety depended on them; they were in control, yet I was responsible. I felt tight, like I was a prisoner of their actions because I was responsible. I was angry at them. I was yelling at them. But nobody was listening.

– *How does it feel to be a prisoner?*

– Scary. It is the question of life and death. It is scary on that level.

– *Describe it more.*

– It felt like I was going to die if they did not give me the wheel. It felt like we were all going to die in the car. It was absurd that I was supposed to be responsible when they were driving. It felt impossible to work it out.

– *Say more about the prisoner.*

– In general, being in my family as a child felt like being a prisoner. It is a feeling like there is no place I can go where I am not gonna feel scared. A place where I can breathe, I can rest, I can enjoy myself, where it is okay for me to trust that things would be okay, and it is okay to be curious, okay to be open.

– *Say more about the prisoner.*

– It feels like I shut all the pores of my skin. If I do not do that I am going to die. I need to do that to protect myself. Wherever it is coming from, it hurts.

– *What is coming that hurts?*

– If I do not shut everything, anything that will be open will result in me being hurt. I cannot take it anymore. I experience it in all my relationships with my family. Whatever I do I feel not appreciated.

– *Say a little more about this.*

– I am a prisoner of myself. I have to do that bubble. It is a state of survival. I go there to protect myself because everything else around me I experience as dangerous. But I also feel trapped.

> This is the equal opposite aspect of the bubble – when the safe place turns into a prison. A place that she cannot leave because she is scared.

– I would like to go out in the world because I am curious, but I am not able to because I am afraid.

– *Tell me more about shutting the pores.*

– In a situation where in my family I would go to one of them, then to the other, then to the other, then to the other. I realize I can go nowhere. Wherever I go I will not have connection, compassion, and any interaction that will make me feel better. Then I feel there is no hope. I feel in danger. So I shut it closed. It is a question of life and death. When I get to this point it is extreme. I shut the pores in order to survive. That was my coping.

– *Tell me more about the fact that you did not belong.*

– I wanted to belong more than anything else. My family did not provide that stability. I wanted to look for an identity in a culture. Wanted to belong to a group. I bounced from one group to the other. I did not build attachments.

> Oxygen, as an element, readily creates bonds with other elements. We also breathe through our skin, our pores, not only through our lungs. At the time of this interview, in 2004, my understanding of this row was very rudimentary. The exact differentiation between the remedies was not yet clear. But I knew that she needed a mineral remedy from the row of the periodic table that corresponded to the stages of birth, describing the process of detaching from the source. This recognition was strengthened by the fact that she was talking about the bubble as a safe, protective place around her, and detachment from her family. Since she used the word oxygen as something she needed in ways that did not make a lot of sense, I thought it must carry some importance to the case. She also mentioned not being able to breathe, of suffocating and choking, a few times during the interview.
>
> About the effects of smoking on one's health we know that the poisonous gas, carbon monoxide is present

in cigarette smoke, and the capacity of blood to carry oxygen is diminished by the carbon monoxide that binds to hemoglobin much more readily than oxygen, causing heavy smokers' blood deprived of oxygen. This kind of information becomes relevant as we are searching for the relationship between the substance the remedy is made of and the words people use to describe their situation. In Fanny's case cigarette smoke takes over the role of oxygen, just as carbon monoxide takes over the role of the oxygen molecules in binding to hemoglobin.

At the first follow-up, four weeks after taking the remedy, Fanny tells me:

– Two things happened: I cried a lot. I cried every day after the remedy. I cried about my sister who died. I felt down, depressed. But I moved through what I was feeling.

– *What do you mean by that?*

– I will get upset but then I can move through what I am feeling. I can move through my feelings. The other interesting thing that happened is that the cigarettes have a different taste now. It is a taste I remember from the time I was a teenager. It is a cinnamon flavor. It reminds me of a time when I started smoking. I was on the porch of a friend, chewing cinnamon gum and smoking. The rain started pouring. It rained hard. It felt very good.

– *Describe this sensation more.*

– I have a sensation in my throat where I am checking the taste of the cigarettes. I remember checking the cinnamon taste in my throat.

– *Have you ever had it since that teenage experience?*

– I had it once last year. And now, after the remedy.

– *Tell me about that time when you were on that porch.*

– It was an escape. I liked to be alone. But I was sad and lonely. It was a spiritual, existential moment for me. The rain had some cleansing effects on me. I felt it was containing me. I felt connected to the universe, the universe that is bigger than me.

– *Containing?*

> Before Fanny answers this question, she makes the
> gesture of the bubble around her with her hands again.

– Surrounded with nature. I am part of it. I always feel good in a snowstorm. It feels out of control and I am inside it; I am surrounded by it, by this force of nature.

– *Tell me about the crying.*

– I always felt there was no space for me to cry. I cried when my sister died, at the funeral. But since then I have not cried. I feel at peace with that not crying. For me it means having the time. It feels spacious. I was not trying to make the crying happen. Since the remedy I am also angry more spontaneously. I had a big fight with my partner. Becoming angry is my clutch. Because of our son, who we recently adopted, our life is more stressful. One day when he was getting out of control I wanted to put him under a cold shower but my partner did not agree with and put her hand on the faucet. It was enough to trigger me. It affected my control, put me out of safe place.

– *Put you out of safe place?*

– I had a dramatic childhood. I have been traumatized. I had no safe place to exercise my will.

– *Describe the feeling when she put her hand on the faucet.*

– I felt blank. Then I went through all the feelings in three hours. Usually it takes me days. Right now there would be enough reason to struggle. But somehow I am able to go through with it. My partner also says I am not as stuck as before the remedy. I also feel the need to isolate less so I am more extroverted. I am closer to the surface of the water.

– *Have you experienced any return of past symptoms?*

– Yes. When I was 12 my left wrist cracked. It has been hurting now for three weeks! I also feel the back pain exactly where I fell years ago! It has been causing me hip and upper back pain before my periods, but not the very spot I hit it. Now it hurts there.

> Fanny has been improving on the remedy beautifully.
> We can sense a major shift happening along with the

return of the old symptom, which is a positive sign
of the remedy taking effect. Her healing is still in
motion; it has not stopped. The right action at this
time is to wait, not to repeat the remedy. The function
of a remedy is to start the body's own self-healing
mechanism. When in relatively good health, the body
can utilize its own self-healing mechanism. Sometimes,
when the stress on the system is too great the body
needs some help. That is what the homeopathic
remedy provides. Once the mechanism ignited, it
keeps going on its own. There is no need to interfere
with more remedy. In some instances, an impatient
homeopath could in fact halt the healing process by
repeating a remedy too soon. As long as the person is
improving, there is no need to take more doses. This
is a point that is often hard to comprehend for
Western-trained minds. In Western thinking we have
learnt the more the better. This is just one of the
things we have to unlearn when approaching healing
with homeopathy.

Two months later, Fanny comes to see me with her
son and offers a short summary about herself:

– I find flow and I go. It is really helping. I do not get so frozen,
stuck, paralyzed as it would have happened in the past when I had
as much stress as I do right now. I feel so much more grounded. I
panic less. If I am angry I express it right away; I do not hold it
inside. I am less afraid so I just say it. I do not doubt myself as
much. I feel my compassion more. I feel a general flow and much
more breath inside of me. Instead of my feeling clumsy, crooked,
in unbalanced ways, it is just flowing, going. It has a circular motion.
It is just going. There is a sense that it is a forward motion, as
opposed to the past when it would be forward, stop, forward,
stop. I still feel that particular taste of cigarette in my throat.

At another follow-up visit three months later, just
before Christmas, Fanny tells me:

– I feel as though I need more air. I have been observing my breath patterns in my yoga practice and have noticed where it blocks: in the upper chest and mid-lungs. This is also where I experience back pain, and it is also related to my wrist pains, which I am experiencing again. It is no doubt related to my smoking, which I am doing more of since the beginning of the winter and holiday seasons. I also feel more stuck on an emotional level, like I am carrying more and letting go less, and I need to soothe (oral soothing, i. e., smoking) more to get by on a day-to-day basis. And I feel it is increasing, which makes me anxious. This is a restless time for me. Each year I find a way to survive it. I am more disorganized and I sleep less, so I am tired, which in turn makes me even more disorganized. I smoke more, I eat more, I isolate more. I detach myself from the feelings so I can cope with the time. This is a holding on, tightening phase.

> She accompanies this explanation with her fists tight, a pronounced hand gesture. I ask her to describe this.

– I feel like I am going for a ride: I tighten up, take a deep breath and just wait until I get there! Find soothing and just wait it out.
– *Why is it this time of the year?*
– It is probably the combination of different things. Christmas was always a time when there were more fights in my house when I was growing up. This is also the time of the year when I was alone in Paris, trying to come to terms with my childhood and decide how to continue my life. My sister came to visit me and attempted to commit suicide. It was before she was diagnosed with schizophrenia. I was a student, had no money; the school did not help me to figure out how could I help her. I did not know I could ask for help. In Paris I was going through a determining phase when I was realizing my childhood and facing things that happened. I chose to detach myself, to separate completely from the family, so I could heal myself. At work I get angry at the system. I have to be angry. I have no choice. I do not have the power to have the choice to be angry. I don't have a choice! I want to be able to choose how to react to conflict.

— How do you react to this internally?

— I have to detach myself, because it is too personal. I am disorganized. I cannot align myself to their values. It is an abusive power. I feel like a baby that is not in control. There is no hope. It triggers me. I am forced into a position to lie, to pretend. There is chaos, confusion. It is unsafe. There are no guidelines. The other thing that bothers me at work is that there is no connection amongst people who are working together. It is a metaphor for my family. There was definitely no connection between us. It was life in denial. My feelings were taken away from me. When I told my father about my feelings he just brushed me away by saying, "Oh, you are not feeling that!"

— Denial?

— Denial makes me feel powerless. My need for change stems from my wanting to feel that power! So I need to break it apart. But at the moment I feel I do it out of reaction. I would like to do it mindfully.

— Describe that breaking apart.

— Like breaking glass with my fist. Krshttt!

> She gestures with her fist as if breaking glass in front of her and gives a breaking sound.

The denial is the glass and I make it fall.

— Describe the breaking of the glass. How does it feel to break it?

— It's freedom! It is a relief. So I can finally connect to the person who is in denial. I need connection and in order to do that, I need to break it so we can communicate.

> Her language describes breaking away from the source. She does not feel validated, which makes her feel unsafe. Her reaction is anger. This anger causes breaking away. If you switch your perception again you can almost see the atoms and molecules how they need to break and connect. This is a deep level of perception when a person is able to talk in terms of the source of their remedy.

The very words Fanny uses return to the same theme: it is always about being in a whole, in a unit which then breaks and she needs to or is compelled to break away, to remove herself. Think of the baby being born. Having the pressure from the outside and the feeling that she cannot be a part of that environment anymore, she needs to break it. She needs to leave, to break the glass wall; in order to survive she has to get out. The fetus that had such a safe environment starts feeling the pressure; the water needs to be broken and she has to leave. Her very survival would be threatened if she stayed. Her place now is outside of this safe, protected environment.

– *What is your integrity?*
– Honesty towards myself. I need this honesty in my environment to feel safe and also I need to have inner honesty. Growing up I experienced learning mechanisms of how to deny things. My only way to get out of that trap is to make sure I do not get into dishonesty.
– *How does it feel to be safe?*

She takes some time to think about her answer. As a smile spreads on her face, she opens her arms wide and says:

– Surrounded by people that own everything.
– *Own it?*
– Own everything they do, comfortable with who they are. Even if I get mad with them they are still comfortable. It gives me hope that I can navigate towards truth. It gives me hope that I won't be stuck, that I won't feel I cannot move even if I feel I am shrinking, suffocating, or if I feel I am not going anywhere. I am not imprisoned. I am free to go if I feel I cannot do this.

After this visit, Fanny takes one dose of Oxygen 200c, and I do not see her for twelve months. Then she brings her son in for treatment. She tells me that she has not been getting colds at all since taking Oxygen.

Once she repeated it because her old wrist pain was
surfacing again. She was very happy with the results.
As she talks about herself she shows a curious, new,
spiral-shaped gesture with her hands. I ask her to come
in for a visit. I want to explore this hand gesture. Next
week she comes in:

– I saw a healer last week that works with the concept called
"uncording" yourself. It means that instead of the umbilical cord
kind of relationship you try to connect to others by other means,
like from the heart, spiritually, or professionally.

I find this "coincidence" intriguing. Fanny's
homeopathic remedy comes from the second row of
the periodic table, the very essence of which is the
release from the womb, the birth process. This is
another example of how we are drawn to things and
people in our lives that correspond to our energetic
makeup. Fanny no doubt has been touched by this
particular practice. Noting that she is being influenced
by the healer, I have to be aware that she will use
language that derived from the healer and not mistake
it for her own words. On the other hand, the way she
describes the healer's work or the terminology she
repeats is in some way related to her. Everything she
relates about others is in some way expresses her own
inner reality. This idea will be expressed in other case
examples: all we perceive is mirroring our inner self.
Thus, we as homeopaths can include all that into our
consideration for a remedy choice.

– I was stronger than my parents so I "fed" or "corded" them.
My whole family was all in great need of being fed with someone's
energy. I took on the role to do that while I would not get
anything in return. So I learned to nurture myself through music
and art. When I realized that I was nurturing myself so I could
nurture them, I stopped. I did not want to nurture them. And I
am still stuck in it today: I am not able to sing. I would love to

have a gig and I would love to paint, but whenever I start I get anxious, I cannot do it. I am carrying my childhood fear today. It is blocking me from being strong, good in something. My fear is that if I become strong, their cords will automatically come and attach to me. It is preventing me from growing up.

– Describe these cords.

– I imagine myself as an octopus with long hands. I am very talented with these hands. I reach out with them. I achieve things with them. I think it is a strength to be able to work these arms. But there are people at the other end attached to these cords. And they are sucking out of me. Draining out of me. As an adult I have learned to reject what I do not want but it takes a lot of energy. At the same time I am afraid to cut these cords because I am scared to be alone, abandoned, lonely. On one hand I know I need to nurture myself so I need to cut those cords but the transition is hard.

– Transition is hard. You are afraid to be lonely, abandoned?

– The dominant thing is that I am scared to do the thing that makes me happy. If I do, something bad is going to happen. My parents are not going to talk to me. My sister will not talk to me. They will hate me for it.

> Fanny dreads being disconnected. As an example she always brings up her family members. When she is talking about having people at the other end of the cords she mentions that they are draining from her. She does not want that. But on the other hand she is afraid to let go of the connection because she would lose the family members' close attachment. She feels drained by it but scared to let go.

– I am also afraid that maybe I am wrong. I am afraid once I realize I made a mistake, that it is not for me, I cannot go back anymore.

> This is where Fanny experiences hesitation, the fear of being ready to leave but being afraid of letting go. This is the theme that symbolizes the actual process

of leaving the womb, going through the birth canal and emerging into the world and taking the first breath of life. This is definitely a turning point: there is no way back, you have to let go.

– Fear is my strongest emotion.
– *How does fear feel in your body?*
– It is a terror in my body. Great sadness. I cannot connect to anybody. The fear is choking me. I am enraged and desperate. I feel helpless. I feel I am in an ocean, the currents are trying to shove me down and I want to fight back. I know I have to reach a distant island. Eventually I let myself down.
– Recently I painted a painting: it expresses my relationship to my mother. It is spiral red. I was enraged. The circle got bigger when I was painting that. Then when I was drawing the bigger and bigger circles I was flooded with love, as opposed to the small circles in the beginning, when I was suffocating inside me. I felt beautiful and powerful.

> You can almost see the birthing of this baby that emerges from the mother, with all the mixed emotions. Eventually the storm calms down and she feels loved again. The beginning starts with pressure from the surroundings as she describes it in so many ways. It also expresses itself as pressure in her head, in the collar bone – pressing physical symptoms. Then swimming in the water that has a strong undercurrent. Then eventually she feels calm again.

– Rage is my coping. I have fifteen paintings like that. On the surface I am frozen, unable to move towards my safety but inside it is very alive. Nobody knows it is moving inside. I need to let it out. It is a scary place. I need to communicate to the outside world. It looks like a tunnel, a scary place.
– *Describe that scary place.*
– I see myself in a room breaking everything, taking knives, stabbing pillows. In the eye of the tornado nothing can get to me. I am safe. It is a place where I go and nobody can hurt me.

This is the bubble. I do not talk when I am there. I am not verbal. I isolate myself. I don't want to be bothered. I used to be in that state for days, but now it's a maximum two hours.

This is expected once she has taken a few doses of her homeopathic remedy that corresponds to her inner world.

– *You mentioned feeling abandoned earlier.*

– If someone wants something from me, I feel the urge to give, I cord people. I cannot ignore them, probably because I do not want to feel abandoned. I do not need it now but I am prone to being addicted to it. This ties in the addiction to smoking. Smoking is creating the protective bubble around me.

– *Opposite of being abandoned? What do you lose?*

– I lose my tribe, my root, identity, where I come from, my grounding.

– *What do these words stand for?*

– Survival. After not talking to my parents for a year I will call them, connect to them. Even if it is not easy for me I have to tap into it again, because I know that is where the answer is.

At the end of this visit, Fanny receives another dose of Oxygen. The reason for repeating the same remedy is that she is still describing the same inner sensation: the need for disconnection from the family, the addiction and attachment to the safe bubble, and because it has been helping her.

A month later, Fanny sends me an email:

I think this remedy helps me a lot to move through my feelings and have less fear in terms of expressing them. I feel generally more lighthearted and can more easily let go of things. I feel less angry. But I keep getting sick with colds and sinus infections, and I don't want to take any more antibiotics because obviously they don't work.

In two months she comes for a follow-up visit:

– I am here today because the last two or three years I have been getting sick a lot: colds mainly, but in general since I moved to North America I have not been well. I have had seasonal allergies, psoriasis and these colds. I have not mentioned it before but now I feel I need to take this extra step to be really healthy. The remedy has really helped with my emotions but not with the colds. Before the remedy I had trouble expressing myself. At home I can explain myself but as soon as I go out in the world I start doubting myself. Since the remedy I have been much better in this sense. A few times I was really surprised, even shocked at how easily I handled normally stressful conflict situations. It is so much simpler now. I don't hang onto my feelings. I am able to express them. Getting sick is a good excuse not being in the world.

– *Getting sick is a good excuse?*

– It keeps me partly safe, partly unhappy. Because I don't do anything. I shut down. There is a lot of pressure and tension in the head and even in the ears. When I'm sick I feel helpless, powerless and vulnerable.

– *What is the opposite of this feeling?*

– A sense of community, when we talk openly, transparently. That is my strength, that is where I shine. I remember having a sense of community with my girlfriends in Japan. I had a sense of belonging. It gave me energy, power.

– *What is energy and power?*

– A state of no ego. That is what I associate with community.

> Notice that when she is sick her problem is the lack of energy and powerlessness. She describes connection to a community as characterized by power and energy. So when she is sick she misses the connection. We are back again to the basic theme, her innermost experience. Her answer also reveals that her natural state is lack of ego. The development of ego is a theme of the third row of the periodic table. Thus, the first two rows have not developed their egos yet. The state of community, of her personal protecting bubble, where she feels she belongs (i. e., to a source) is her most natural state. It is an egoless state.

– *Last time you mentioned the tornado. How is it doing?*

– The difference from last time is that I feel okay in the eye. I am protected there and I do not feel that I am losing control.

She gestures with a twirly motion of her hand.

– There can be danger all around but if I stay there I won't be swept around. I used to be in the tornado. Now, as I am sitting there in the center of the tornado I feel I have a voice, that I am there by choice. I am aware that this is a coping that works for me. In my office everything is out of control. I feel trapped and scared. Before we started homeopathic treatment I used to quit my job in situations like this. Now I stay. I don't need to run away now.

> Six months later, Fanny reports that she has not had a cold or sinus problem since the last dose of the remedy.

A CASE OF ECZEMA

Once completely separated from the source, individuals arrive at the next step of development: creating an identity for themselves. This is the third line of the periodic table, where the ego emerges – a phase that is healthy and normal for young children. They exercise their identity, first by declaring that a toy belongs to them. Then, later they establish their own self as a person that others should listen to instead of brushing them aside, saying they are too young to understand. While we would not prescribe a remedy based on these issues to a child, as for them it is a healthy developmental stage, if an adult is concerned with expressions of their ego development and not able to step beyond it, they might benefit from a homeopathic remedy prepared from a mineral found in this row.

Remedies in the next line, the fourth, are concerned with safety. In order to survive in their perceived universe, people need to provide safe shelter for themselves and others. In the beginning of the line, all they have energy to think about is their own protection. But as we go further in the line, we see individuals who are deeply concerned with protecting others as well as being successful in their own protection. There are eighteen elements in this line; thus, the differences will be rather slight. The theme of the next line, the sixth is adventure. Once the previous issues such as safety and security have been resolved, an individual continues to explore their surroundings – the universe – and will see how can it be stretched and improved upon. This is the line the next case comes from.

> Nick is a 44-year-old man suffering from acute flare-ups of eczema. He is polite and well dressed. He tells me he has done various searches on the Internet to get started on this path. He looked up several homeopaths in the area and found my website. He read all the pages and felt comfortable with what he found there.

– *How can I help you?*

– The most immediate issue is the eczema. I have had it since adolescence. It pops up in wintertime. It was fairly manageable until recently, appearing only in the arm bends and behind the knees. It was not pleasant but I could get rid of it with some cortisone. Eight years ago I had a bad flare-up when it went to my face. The doctor put me on two consecutive courses of Prednisone®. Ever since then it keeps coming back, worse and worse each time.

This winter it got out of control. It was on my arms, my chest, my face and neck. I got a higher dose of steroids and got sick from them for three weeks. It lessened the severity of the symptoms but did not cure the eczema. The problem is that the cortisone does not work anymore. I have built up a resistance to it. I was also frustrated that I always got a cream and drugs that gave symptomatic relief. I want to affect my eczema. It seems to be getting worse as I am getting older. I want to approach it in a more holistic manner.

I am an analyst at work, a systems engineer. What I do is, I look at the big picture. I understand that silver-bullet solutions that contractors propose do not work; they do not fix the big problem. You have to treat the system as a whole, work it as a whole. That is what I am not seeing in my medical treatment. I am not being treated as a whole person. When I go to see a dermatologist I narrow it even more down. I want to back up to look at things in a larger perspective.

> Nick's hands start to move as he speaks. A large circular gesture accompanies the idea of the big picture and a different one, where he holds his hands parallel to each other, go with the narrow, compartmentalized thinking.

– *What are the actual symptoms of your eczema?*

– This last flare-up was really bad. The rash was widespread. The worst was after a shower. It felt as if the skin was sandblasted!

– *How does it feel when the skin is sandblasted?*

– It is stinging, painful, and itchy, constantly raw. I was really uncomfortable. Sometimes I had to work from home to stay in less irritating clothes and go to the office only for meetings. I went to Florida last week and it helped a lot. The combination of the sun and moisture made my skin much better. I have been doing a body cleanse. I researched and found a product that cleanses all the organs. I changed my diet and reduced many environmental factors that could contribute to the flare-ups.

> The same big, circular hand gestures accompany his recount of the sun and moisture helping his skin and his change in diet.

– I will back up a little: the other reason I am here is that I want to improve my lifestyle, my health in general. I have started this change by using the cleanse by consciously changing my eating habits. Now I buy organic produce and try to be health conscious in my decisions. We removed all carpets from the house, bought a shower filter that neutralizes chlorine and do other little things like these. I feel I am on a path I like.

– *Tell me more.*

> I do not ask for specifics so that he can say what is on his mind. The questioning style is as open-ended as possible. Often the question is there only to encourage the natural flow of the narrative. The question is not leading into a specific direction, as that would alter the path the person would naturally take.

– I still have these lingering health issues I would like to resolve. It is the eczema that pushed me over the edge, but I feel I had been walking down this path before that. This was what motivated me to look at alternative medicine – taking my health care into my own hands instead of handing it over to someone else.

– *Pushed you over the edge?*

– I have an orthodox science background so it was difficult for me to break out from the scientific method of analyzing and diagnosing to open my horizons a little bit and look at things that did not exactly fit into that worldview where you could get your arms around everything: analyze and feel and see. It has been a good process; it has opened me up a bit. I even went to a meditation class they organized at work There is so much more to it than people know in the Western scientific world. I am feeling more and more comfortable with it. I was on that path anyway. I have spent my last year researching and reading about these things. I had heard about homeopathy before but when the eczema came I thought that was the right time to try it and not to put it aside any longer.

> Here Nick is using the same hand gesture as he did with describing the narrowing down of specialization of dermatology. Both hands parallel to each other bringing them rather close, as opposed to his other characteristic hand gesture: the broad, opening, wide circular motions.
>
> At a later point during the interview I usually ask people to describe their hand gestures. Not the words that accompany them, just the gestures themselves. I ask people to repeat the gesture and report what they feel, what they sense while doing it. Some people are deeply touched by the sensation. Even though for the outsider it might look like a random hand movement, the sensation it evokes touches the person that experiences it. It brings forth sensations that will be general, not just local and specific to their complaint. Once a local sensation becomes general – i. e., repeats itself in the story of the patient – it becomes a general sensation for this person and will bear great importance for the prescriber.

– I like this image of being on the path. Can you say more about it? You told me about it in practical terms but now say more in terms of the image. Describe that.

– Well, it is a good question. Let me think about how to verbalize it.

– *Take your time.*

– It is intertwined: it is a spiritual, intellectual and medical thing at the same time. I am very curious, interested in alternative approaches. I have an intellectual curiosity about many things, life in general. Health-wise I have seen benefits from the changes I made, by stepping away from the commercial culture. The spiritual sense has been intriguing me also for a long time. When I decided to go to the meditation class I had no idea what were we doing. But then I got it. I started feeling some of its physical effects. I am just scratching the surface here obviously, but it has been a progress. There is so much there I do not know. After the meditation class I was relaxed and energized at the same time. It is interesting how you can feel these two at the same time.

– *Tell me more about the relaxed and energized at the same time. How does it feel?*

– Again, I am just scratching the surface here. My mind is always running. I am a planner, an organizer – my mind is always thinking about something. For example, when we go on a vacation I like to research and find out about things we can do there. I enjoy that kind of planning. When I came out of those meditation sessions I did not feel like I was jumping from one thing to the other; I could focus easily. Usually I focus well; but the ease with which I could go from one thing to the other was amazing.

– *Flow from one thing to the other with ease?*

– That is going to be a hard one to describe… What I was able to do coming out of those sessions was being able to very clearly see what I needed to do next. Instead of going through the list I kind of knew what I needed to do next. It is part of that path. It is not like I have dots lined up and I just have to go from one dot to the other but there are lots of dots and I am trying to figure out my way through them, which dot to go to next. There is a goal at the end, maybe, but I don't know if I will ever get there. That is not the point. I just want to get closer. It is not a predetermined path.

– *What is your experience of going from one dot to the other?*

– I am very curious by nature. I explore, I research. Let's say there are stages. The first one is an exploratory stage. If it is something I find interesting I file it somewhere in my mind for later to find out more about it. If it interests me I want to find out the best or a good way to approach it. Then it goes where it goes. The executing part is when I try to change things in my life to fit the new thing in. While I am doing that I am still doing the exploration part as well.

> Mentioning the word *research* several times seems quite significant. Earlier Nick mentioned he had researched the health field and found certain products to help his healthy lifestyle. He said it very soon after describing his chief complaint. That's significant because that is the way he first introduces himself to me. He tells me he spent time and effort researching the available healing modalities, and once he found homeopathy he read everything on my website. While I usually ask people how they found me and often they tell me it was through Internet search, it is rare to hear that one read all the information available on my website. I know I have to wait until this unusual fact fits into the bigger puzzle of Nick's case. While I keep listening to him I note that research bears importance for him. In this last segment he reinforces this aspect in talking about research and exploration. He does not go on to the stages of success or maintaining what he has gained. Those issues are not in the focus of his attention.

– *Let's go back to the skin. You said it felt like sandblasted.*
– Oh, yes. Like when you are on the beach and the strong wind blows the sand.
– *How does that feel?*
– Little stinging, individual small fires. Tiny dots of fire. All up your arms, back and neck. It tends to come up all at once, not a gradual thing. It was pretty intense. Then it would gradually

subside over time. I also have a nut allergy. I had an episode once when I had cookies with Brazil nuts and I had to be rushed to the emergency room. I almost passed out by the time we got there. My throat was closing up; I had a whole body sensation of tingling. A very unnatural feeling. I also have some more minor food allergies, like to scallops.

> He goes on talking about details that are irrelevant to the thread of thoughts that would lead into the realm of sensations. So I ask a question that usually brings about volunteered information that expresses the inner sensation:

— *Do you have dreams?*

— Yes, all kinds of dreams. Most often things that I have done well or could have done better. Or I change the ending so I would do better. I have lots of dreams that are competitive, like sports competitive. I have a competitive side.

— *Talk about that.*

— It is a sports-related competitiveness. I am achievement oriented in management, at work. And it bleeds through to playing sports and games. I love to play cards, love to play games. I love to go to Las Vegas. I love to play Black Jack, Poker, all the card games. I don't like gambling, but I love to play games. I'll play basketball in the driveway. Or give me a hockey stick and put up a net in the driveway. Any kind of game.

— *Tell me what you like in games.*

— The competition. In poker you can lose even with the best hand. It is the question of strategy. You are looking for the pattern — what you can pick up from a partner. As I said earlier I am quite analytical. So I keep asking myself: What can I do to win? It is all about strategy.

— *Tell me more about your experience of competition, winning and strategy.*

— Some people run long distance to feel energized and focused. They are engaged, totally engaged. I play competitive games to achieve the same, to move the endorphins.

— *What do you enjoy in competition?*

– I don't like video games, combat-stimulation. Those are too violent. That is scary to me, too much about death. That deadens you. I don't like betting either. I like competitiveness. Then the game, the match is over. No need to crash cans. That is over the edge. For me the spirit of competition is more evident in sports or work.

– *How successful are you in these things?*

> By now we can see that the main issue for Nick is performance. He competes to sharpen his competitive strategy. It is not about winning over the other as it would be in the animal kingdom. It is about improving his inner ability. This means he needs a mineral remedy. As I mentioned earlier, in mineral cases we have to clarify the person's exact spot in the periodic table. This will be done by understanding which line and which column matches their issues. Nick has been hinting which line he belongs to by his inborn instinct to research and explore new, uncharted areas. This is the theme for the fifth row of the periodic table.
>
> The next step is to understand where, in which column on that line, he is, which stage of development is the most challenging for him. That is why I ask the question how successful he is. He has been describing exploration and working towards a goal that fits the beginning of the development we see throughout a line of the periodic table. When he describes the path of dots he says he knew there was a goal but for him the important thing was that he was on the way towards that goal, not the actual goal. This places him somewhere on the left side of the column, before the peak in success, which would be the middle point of the line. He says he was scratching the surface, again a phrase that hints the beginning stages.

– In poker I am not going to be on TV soon. I am good at things I get serious about. When you learn strategies, they carry over. For example, I loved coaching basketball. I love the game; it is fun.

– *Fun?*

– It is fun because it is out of the box, unconventional. It is about a willingness to try things. There is also a strong social component to it: getting people together in a casual setting. To relax together, to play, to have fun. Not just work. I am trying to explore what we can achieve if we relate to each other differently. I always wanted to get people out of the work environment. Playing together is one idea. My love for basketball comes from high school when I played on the team, but more recently I have coached my kids' team. I love the coaching aspect of the game.

– *Tell me about coaching.*

> I need to grasp which aspect of coaching is meaningful for him. There are many elements in each activity. The activities themselves will not determine the categories a person can be said to belong to; it is the inner experience that counts. Just because Nick likes coaching does not mean that he will need the same remedy as another coach. From what Nick says it is clear he enjoys the teaching, which is a characteristic of the fifth row. We can also say that he is not one of the first remedies on the row because those people feel so inadequate in the discovering of new things that they would not be able to coach others. You need a certain degree of self-assurance to coach others. The group of remedies he might need is getting narrower: he is on the left side of the fifth row but not the very first ones. As he talks further, he describes his exact inner experience, which places him on an exact spot on this row.

– In a game I am assessing the other team: their size, their quickness. I am matching up what they can do. I am looking at what kind of offense and defense they have and then trying to adapt in real time. Exploit the other team. It is like puzzles. Game.

You fully engage. You are trying to win the game. I am teaching the kids to play the best they can play.

— The best they can play?

— They always have to check in with themselves: Am I playing my best? It is self-competition. I am not competing with the others. It is all about me. Am I learning, am I getting better? Can I rise up to the challenge? Can I overcome my weaknesses? As a coach it is my job to put my team into the best position. I do the best I can. It is an internal competition.

> Nick uses the same large, circular hand gesture again. At this time his hands keep moving in large circles with a lot of emphasis. This is a crucial part of the case. After he describes what competition means for him, he confirms to me that he needs a mineral remedy. The hand gesture that accompanies a statement shows that the utterance is meaningful for him on the energetic level as well.

— Tell me about this hand gesture.

> He pauses while moving his hands in the same fashion and looking inward to find the answer to the question.

— Things are in motion. Life is not static; life is in motion. Stuff is going on in the real world. Everything is changing all the time. We and everything else is physically growing up, changing. My company is changing. It involves corporate strategy. The question is where we are trying to get. Everything is evolving, moving on. It is invigorating to live in a time when things are changing. I like it that way. People call it risk. I call it opportunity. And I see it not only in my job but also in my family life. My son was born with disabilities. I see this as an opportunity for growth. He is the best thing that ever happened to me. I learn so much from the experience with him.

> At this point, Nick goes on to describe an experiment of how for the first time he had eye contact with his son. He watched what his son was doing for a while

(banging kitchen cabinets). Once he had detected the pattern his son was "working" with, he also started doing the same thing. This action on his part clicked something in his son's mind and he looked at his father. This was an amazing moment. Eye contact was not something he shared a lot with people!

This little story also verifies Nick's interest in experimenting and his analytical approach. Not only does it confirm mineral kingdom, it also confirms again and again issues of the fifth line, the line of learning new things, research, creativity. People on the fifth line are often pioneers in their field. They are the ones who do not hesitate to take risks. They thrive on the challenge and love learning, exploring. The other side of the coin is that they also like teaching. They are great coaches who challenge their pupils, just as they challenge themselves.

The particular spot on the fifth row has to do with growth, not with decline. Nick is teaching his students to be the best they can be.

– *Tell me about the change. How far are you in the process?*

– I am at the beginning. I wish I had started it a long time ago. Physically, I am an adult. But spiritually, emotionally, I am just starting to grow up. I am 43… I was very rigid growing up. I started to tear that wall down intentionally. I am not yet nearly where I want to be. But I am willing to do it. Keep moving forward and not let life pass by. I used to be very passive. People would say he is a "nice guy." I never made any waves. But then when my kids were born they had health issues. I had to step up. I understood that I could be assertive and a nice guy at the same time. I changed my personality. I used to be shy. I realized that I could still be quiet but assertive. I could stand up for myself. I had to. I knew my kids better than the doctors. It took me thirteen years to figure it out about myself! I know I am not a fast learner!

He laughs.

But I will certainly get there. For your question, how far I am —
well, I don't think I am real far down the path. I grew up Catholic.
Then I started having problems with the church. I was in a
marriage that was not working. I just let things slide, swept things
under the rug.

When I became more assertive, I made the decision: my marriage
was not working. The spiritual part was missing. I moved to a
different church and got remarried. I am truly happy now. I can
see the benefits from not being passive, from not just letting
things go. I am trying to make some strides. I have seen that and
it is self-reassuring! But I need help and I am not afraid to admit
it. I need help and I am willing to seek it. I am looking forward
to side poles along the way! I believe that we are not put here by
ourselves. It is probably for a reason.

> Here he pauses. Nick is eloquently describing where
> he is on the silver line. He was born in a situation
> where he did not question, did not challenge his
> situation. He was going along, letting life pass by. But
> at a certain point he developed an urge to be more
> proactive: speak up and learn about his own life,
> improve his situation by not accepting it but actively
> seeking to change it. He says he is still quite at the
> beginning. But then he describes how he has changed
> and we realize that he has gone quite a distance. He
> has been continuously challenging himself, building
> himself up. He is not afraid to admit that he needs
> help along the way. People in the beginning of the
> silver line are encouraged by challenging situations,
> and do not shy away from looking for help and
> support from others. Nick has worked his way up to
> this point and he does not stop. Let's see where he
> brings us further in the case:

– In sports I am being challenged. Again, it is not so much the
winning or losing. But a sport is a total body immersion. At
work I am challenged, too. I am paid to think. I like to be

intellectually challenged at work. But it is not the complete whole body challenge as in sports. Even when I am coaching it is a whole body immersion. You are in it in a much more active way than at work.

— What does the word challenge mean for you?

> I ask a question like this when I hear the same word repeating itself over and over again. At this point Nick is spontaneously talking about his passion, his hobby. During this part in the interview people usually get animated: they use body and hand gestures to show how they feel inside. This is the meeting point of body and energy. This is where we can see the remedy. If we encourage people to tell us how it feels to be in their body right at that moment, they can recount very meaningful things about their true nature. Usually people do not think about the energies that drive their lives. But these energies are there all the time. And where else would it be more prominent than when we fully enjoy what we are doing? Nick is telling me about his love for sports and coaching. He is looking for words to convey what is it that truly matters to him. This is a level that is not about feelings. He is not telling me that he feels good about himself or feels satisfied. He tells me about his inner experience. It is the sensation that he relates to life with. It is a short cut to the true core of the person.
>
> Asking Nick about what challenge means for him, I hope to hear what type of situation is the one that he struggles with. Translating it to our terms, we will hear which remedy he needs from the more than a dozen remedies on the silver line.
>
> Nick thinks for a second…

— Good question! To me, challenge means that there is some higher level that you are trying to get to and you are not there yet. And it may be one or twenty-seven levels higher. I don't know. But some level you are trying to get to in terms of performance, execution, concentration and creativity. Whatever it is. A mix of those. A higher state you are trying to attain. And it is an internally fueled desire. It is not an external pressure or expectation that somebody has put on you. I don't coach for a living. There is no monetary pressure, or public criticism kind of pressure. It is all internally motivated. A desire on my part to do well, to get to that next level. You always encounter situations that you never encountered before. The question is how you deal with them.

– *When challenged, do you need help or do you feel you can do it all by yourself?*

– It works both ways. Some things I can do by myself. Some things I clearly need help with. I used to be afraid to ask. Now I ask when I need to. That's part of being more assertive.

> This is the information I gathered during the first interview. It boils down to the remedy made from the eighth element in the silver line: Technetium. This remedy is a new addition to a homeopath's repertoire. Before the use of the periodic table to understand remedies based on the line and the column their source is found in, we could not have prescribed remedies like Technetium. Jan Scholten was the first homeopath to introduce the idea of deducting qualities of unknown remedies based on their location in the periodic table. His book, *Homeopathy and the Elements*, was a groundbreaking step in the evolution of homeopathy. He is the first author who mentions Technetium (among many other new remedies). According to his understanding Technetium is on the line of creativity. The seventh column stands for the developmental stage of practicing one's skills, fine-tuning and cooperating with others.
>
> Scholten says of Technetium: "…they know they are on the right track. Compliments stimulate their

ambitions, stimulate them to keep following their chosen path. But they are not averse to criticism either, as long as it is constructive. At least it will show them what adjustments to make to get even better results."[6] (Further understanding of the rows and columns describes Technetium as a person who is an adventurer, a researcher, one who creates something new. He knows he can do it. he has passed the stages of self-doubt but is wondering how far he can manage to go by himself. He looks for allies; people who help him stay on the right track. Thus, in terms of health, the point where a person needing Technetium gets stuck is the stage where they are on their path to succeeding in creating their dreams. They are just about to feel fully successful but usually they sense that something is still missing. They could still improve in order to be satisfied with their achievements. Technetium is three columns before the midline, which is characterized by success. From the midpoint on, issues will be losing that ability for successful creativity and performance or hard work in order to maintain that success. The remedies before the midline are optimistic and are working towards achieving a goal. Technetium is among these remedies, being the eighth in the row.

This is the right remedy for Nick because his inner sensation shows his main concern is about building a successful strategy to win, to better himself and the world around him. When he talks about his family, his main concern is not about their safety as a father from the fourth line would talk about. Rather, he talks about his son's well-being and development. This points to a slightly different attitude in his value

---

[6] Scholten, Jan, *Homeopathy and the Elements*. Utrecht, The Netherlands: Stichting Alonnissos (1996) p. 572.

system, which is conformed in different areas of his life. The specific spot on the line is not always easy to pinpoint. Nick fits the Technetium picture in that he has found a path he walks and works hard at it to keep going on it. He does not mind asking for help. In fact, he feels he needs some guidance to stay on his self-chosen path. His spirit of competition places him on this spot of striving to achieve his goals. He is a competitor, not against another person but rather against himself. He is always eager to prove he can do better. He knows he can do it; thus, he needs a remedy beyond the sixth column where the main concern is doubting their own abilities and feeling that it is such a challenge to work for their goals. Nick knows he can do it. It comes to him naturally to work towards his goals. In the eighth column, perseverance is the most important thing, and in the ninth it is about perfecting and avoiding last-minute glitches. Nick is not concerned with those issues. Neither is he concerned with maintaining his success, feeling that his past glory is escaping him. If this were the case he would need a remedy from beyond the tenth column. Nick takes the remedy in 30c potency. Since homeopathic remedies might aggravate ongoing conditions, a higher potency would have risked a worsening of his eczema, which is best to be avoided. It is a good idea to assess a person's vital strength – their ability to react to a healing remedy – and proceed cautiously to start a gentle healing process without much turmoil. An aggravation, sometimes called a healing crisis, might be inevitable, but if we have the tools to avoid it we have to use them.

I ask Nick to put a dose in water and sip it daily. After a week he reports there is no change in his condition. That is when I tell him to take a dry dose.

First follow-up visit, four weeks later:

– During the first week nothing happened. The second week, right after taking the dry dose, was a rough week. The rash on my arms was painful; it stung, and my chest was itching. Then the following week was easier. By now the patches around my eyes have cleared up and the skin is not as flaky as before. My neck is better; that is the spot that usually gets the worst in the beginning of a flare-up. Right now the worst spot is the top of my wrist; that is my oldest patch.

– *Have you noticed any other change beside the skin?*

– I have never been a morning person. Now in the mornings I feel I rested, ready to go. I even started exercising in the morning. Before I could sleep until noon.

– *Anything else?*

– I must tell you that it was not easy for me to come to see you in the first place. At work my job is to think outside of the box, but it is so different from actually getting out of the box and doing the motions. Being an engineer, homeopathy was not a familiar concept for me.

> As we expand on his comment, he tells me about several "outside the box" activities he has found and has learned to appreciate and incorporate in his life. At later appointments his skin kept improving. The patches spread from his neck and torso over his shoulder, and, as they moved down his arms, the patches on the face, neck and torso disappeared. In May he told me the rash was more superficial; even where it was still present, it did not peel so deeply. After taking one of the doses that helped stop his relapse, he noticed that he had heavy dandruff for a day, the way he had it in high school: "It was as if it was snowing from my head. The next day it was gone." These two phenomena are typical reactions to well-chosen homeopathic remedies. Symptoms such as skin rashes or arthritis tend to move from the center outward

and down on the body. Often the wrist or ankles are the last places these complaints appear, and then they leave for good. The other development, the return of old symptoms, is a similar phenomenon When it happens, old symptoms come back briefly, as if to say goodbye before they move out from the body. These are signs that the illness is moving outwards as opposed to a suppressive therapy where ailments go inside and, even if they become invisible, might lead to chronic consequences of the ill. When we hear reports like this we know the cure is on the right track.

Four months after Nick's initial visit, and taking approximately one dose each month, he tells me that the only two places he had some eczema was the elbow bend and the wrist, the two oldest spots he has had since he was a kid.

– The most important thing I can say about my skin in general is that it feels like normal skin again. Another thing is that I started looking at things in a different light. I always had to-do-lists and never had enough time to accomplish them all. I always did the high pay-off things. Now I looked at my list and suddenly I felt differently about it. It felt like a load was taken off my shoulders. I realized that I started looking and ordering things whether or not I wanted to do them. I feel better up here (points to his head). I feel more energized about the things I do.

On another note, I have been allergic to animals, to mold, and have had some seasonal allergies in the spring and fall. This spring I had no allergies. Zero. As a kid I took antihistamines like candy. Now, after the heavy rains we have had, I was surprised that I did not get any symptoms. About the animal fur I can say that since taking the remedy I visited some friends' who have a dog and usually I last there only half an hour to an hour. After that I start sneezing; I have a fit for 15 minutes. This time I lasted for 2.5 hours and even after that it was maybe two sneezes, that's it. I used to get asthmatic reactions, wheezing, if people came to our house and had their pets' fur on their clothing. That is why I got my inhaler. I have not used it now for a long time.

Now I am like a normal person! I can breathe. I can go to people's houses. Before, in every jacket pocket I had antihistamines. Every time I went somewhere I had to have it… Now I don't. I don't have to. I am much freer to live my life. It's nice. It feels really good.

> Leaving a case on such a positive note is what we aim at with our prescribing. Not only Nick's eczema improved but also a positive process started throughout his organism. The goal of treatment is to achieve a state of health when the person is able to freely manifest his or her true purpose in life. In order to reach that level of being we need good health in body, mind, and spirit. Stories like Nick's suggest that homeopathic treatment is capable of aiding a person in that journey.

I AM NOT A BABY: A CASE OF AUTISM

Amanda, a sixth-grade girl, was diagnosed with autism spectrum disorder when she was two years old. Her mother brings her to see me with the hope that her attention difficulties could ease without using conventional medication. Amanda has been taking Ritalin® and Concerta® since entering first grade. We agree that I will first see Amanda alone, so I can get an impression of her. Then I will meet her mother to fill in the details.

In my session with Amanda, her answer to most of my questions is a short "I don't know." In fact, almost all of her answers tend to be short, and there is a certain suddenness to the way she utters them. I need to repeat my question to hear anything more. This is the underlying energy presenting itself in her manner of speech, and it's important information that I could not have received without seeing Amanda in person. Nevertheless, the most important details of her story are conveyed by her mother. Amanda is at the so-called high functioning end of the autism spectrum disorder. Many children with autism are not able to speak at all or their language is very limited along with characteristic delayed development of social interactions. For some, symptoms can be very similar to those of ADD (Attention Deficit Disorder). Talking to Amanda gives me the opportunity to hear and see the level of her communicational skills, verbal and non-verbal

– *Do you know why your mom brought you here?*
– No.
– *She told me you had been taking Ritalin®. Do you know why?*
– I don't know.
– *Do you feel any difference when you take it or when you don't?*
– Same.
– *I also heard that you have an allergic reaction to peanuts.*
– I don't know. I don't eat peanuts.
– *Let's talk about school. How is school?*
– Good.

– *What grade are you in?*

– Sixth grade.

– *What are your favorite subjects?*

– History. Ancient civilizations.

– *What about friends? Do you have friends?*

– Yes. A lot.

– *Tell me about them.*

– They are nice. I talk to them a lot.

– *What are your hobbies?*

– Hanging out with friends.

– *What else?*

– Doing arts and crafts.

– *Do you have brothers and sisters?*

– A baby sister. I like to play with her.

– *What do you play with her?*

– I play; I babysit her.

– *What do you do with her?*

– Watch TV. But I don't watch anything for her age.

– *Why?*

– Too babyish.

– *What does that mean?*

– Only for little kids.

– *How old are little kids?*

– Like kindergarteners. I don't like to watch shows for her age.

– *Why?*

– Because I already know that stuff they are teaching.

– *What kind of stuff?*

– Like the ABCs.

– *What is for your age?*

– The Princess Diaries.

– *Tell me about it.*

– It is a fantasy. A girl is gonna be a princess. She becomes a princess. It is hard for her. She takes princess lessons. They sound boring.

– *What else do you like doing?*

– I like talking on the phone. I get to spend a long time on it.

– *Who do you talk to?*

– To my friends.

– *Tell me about them.*

– They are nice. They are not mean.

– *Who are mean people?*

– Not sensitive, not nice people. Bad people.

– *Describe them.*

– They say mean things.

– *What kind of things?*

– I don't know what they say about me. That's it.

– *What do they say about other people?*

– I don't know. I don't pay attention to those things.

– *What else do you like doing?*

– I like to look at magazines: *Discovery Girls.*

– *What do they write about in* Discovery Girls?

– Friendships… Am I allowed to drink in here?

> She is asking for my permission to drink. Even though
> I see many children in my office I am not used to
> questions like this. Her asking for my permission
> shows her uncertainty about herself as a decision-
> maker. At this point of the interview I do not draw
> conclusions about the reason behind her question; I
> just make a note of it. Later, I make sure that I take
> this into consideration when analyzing the whole case,
> and see if it fits the rest of the picture.

– *Sure, it's okay to drink. Tell me about things you get excited about.*

– Going to camp. Summer vacation. Other vacations. Breaks.

– *Why breaks?*

– Because there is no school.

– *Tell me about school.*

– I don't like my cluster. I don't like my science teacher.

– *How come?*

– He treats us like babies.

– *How does he treat you like babies?*

– He is asking things like, "What's on the paper?"
– *Why is that treating you like babies?*
– Because we know what's on the paper.
– *Tell me, what would you like to achieve? What would make you feel good to achieve?*
– I want to be good at math.
– *Tell me more about that.*
– I forget everything all the time.
– *How would it feel to be good at math?*
– Good. But I got a lot of math homework last year.
– *And?*
– I am bad at it. I want to be better.
– *Why do you want to be good at math?*
– I want to pay taxes.

> This answer comes out of the blue. These kinds of answers, the ones that mostly surprise us, are the key to the real essence of the case. She has a reason why paying taxes is so important for her. It might not be a conscious reason, so we need to find the way to uncover its roots.

– *How come?*
– I want to be able to do that. Because I want to be a grown-up. Pay for my own things. Use a credit card.
– *How would that feel to do that?*
– I would feel like an adult.
– *How do you think adults feel like?*
– They can do anything by themselves.
– *What else?*
– They have kids. They have jobs.
– *Do you know what would you like to do?*
– No, I don't know.

> In Amanda's mind, adults are able to do things that she is not able to. In order to locate her remedy we need to find out what it is that she can do and what it

is that she cannot. At this point of the interview she is in the right attitude to say what is really on her mind and spontaneously tell me how she sees her abilities. This is what is going to match with her remedy. Her inner sensation about her developmental stage locates her exact spot in our system.

— *What can you do on your own?*
— I can buy bagels. Went once.
— *What else can you do on your own?*
— I can read a book. I can clean my room. I can go on the computer. Do my science homework.
— *What can you not do on your own?*
— Read hard books, like *Long Way from Chicago*. I cannot understand it. We take turns with my mom to read it.
— *What else do you need help with?*
— The DVD player. It is hard to turn it on. I don't even try, because then I end up breaking it. I haven't done it before. I don't know how to do it.

This part of the conversation summarizes Amanda's core sensation. She is incapable of doing things on her own; she needs help. She is not satisfied with this state of dependence on others; she wants to be a responsible grown-up and be able to take care of herself and her kids. She wants to be able to go and buy things. But for now all she can do is buy bagels and read simple books.

Later, Amanda's mom comes in and tells me about Amanda's history:

— She seemed to be developing fine in her first year, but fell apart by the second year. Was it the MMR vaccine? I don't know. By the time she was two and a half we knew something was wrong. Then, after aggressive early intervention, she gradually came back to this life. They diagnosed her with lazy brain syndrome.
— *What do you mean by "fell apart"?*

– She had bad tantrums; she lost whatever words she had had before then. She could not say at the age of three years what she was saying at age of nine months. Language comprehension was not there. She had good cognitive skills. She had tantrums for hours, to a degree where she would stop breathing. She would be banging her head.

– *Tell me about her fears.*

– She used to have very specific fears but she does not have them now. She used to be afraid of long corridors and things like that. Everything had to be taught – both socially and language-wise. What's hot, what's cold, everything.

– *What else can you tell me about her?*

– She is extremely sensitive to criticism. She thinks people are speaking about her, saying bad things about her. If I criticize her, she can blow up; she has extreme reactions, like a five-year-old. She will react to any criticism.

– *You told me she had been on medication.*

– Yes. We put her on Concerta® to improve her attention. Right now we need to increase her dose, I think. She is spacey even though she takes it regularly. It used to help her, but it also made her irritable; everything would trigger her. She would torture us for days with irritability, and irritability is not her personality. I think it is the effect of the drug. We kept giving her the medications because she could concentrate better while taking them, but they also impacted her socially – she is less social when on medication. She says she has lots of friends, but that is not true. Maybe she wants it but she is not very social and others do not want to socialize with her. She would not call any of her friends on the phone. I have to remind her and nag her to call; she does not initiate. She has two friends: one of them has ADD and the other has learning disabilities. She does not make new friends. We have to face it: she is boring for them because she does not talk.

– *What does she do on her own?*

– She can spend hours in her room. She is very passive.

– *Does she have any fears now?*

She is petrified of heights. She is also clumsy; she will not climb, does not have enough coordination. She is extremely poorly coordinated. She walked at eleven months; she was not late with that.

– *What about allergies?*

She is allergic to eggs, soy, and Amoxicillin®. She was throwing up from the first baby food she got.

– *Is she sensitive to being considered a baby?*

> I ask this question because in talking to Amanda the most energetic answer I got from her was regarding her not wanting to watch the TV shows that her baby sister would watch. She also disliked school because of her teacher, against whom her only complaint was that he treated them like babies.

– Yes! She is acting like a five-year-old; she *is* a baby. She does not watch Barney with her little sister because someone might think she is a baby. She would not go to the park with her; she would not play with her toys. She says it is babyish. She is very sensitive to this issue; she is really concerned that others might think she is enjoying baby-like things.

– *How was your pregnancy?*

– Typical, normal thirty-nine weeks, nothing interesting. Some of Amanda's difficulties resemble my late husband's. He was an extremely talented, brilliant engineer but struggled with the most basic language. He would spell phonetically and read slowly. He was exceptionally good in math and science. He was outgoing, always had a lot of friends. He died of a brain tumor when Amanda was five.

– *Tell me about Amanda's way of doing schoolwork.*

– She spends a long time on homework. She can spend one hour just staring at the page without doing anything. On the other hand, she is very good about homework, almost anal. Math provokes her anxiety. She shuts down; she thinks she is not gonna get it. Her writing is very childish; her vocabulary is not mature. She likes to be on stage. Her dancing is terrible – not coordinated

– but she likes it. She quit swimming when she realized she was way bigger than the other kids.

The way to approach the information gathered at the interview is to decide which kingdom Amanda's remedy is from. She is not competitive, as an animal remedy would be, and neither is she sensitive, as a plant remedy would be. It is her inner structure that is the main issue, and her structure is such that she is not capable of living an independent life in this world. The chief complaint is her passivity and delayed development. She started developing fine in her first year of life, then she "fell apart": she stopped developing and regressed. She is capable of basic functions and manages in a regular classroom, even though she needs the help of her aid.

Some key elements in this case point to the remedy, Baryta carbonica. Barium, the element source of this remedy, lies in the intersection of the sixth line and second column of the periodic table. In our previous case we looked into the line of creativity and adventure. As we take a step further, from the fifth to the sixth line, we find that performance is firmly established, and the nature of development leads to responsibility. Issues of the sixth line are around leadership and responsibility. At the beginning of the line there are those who are the most incapable of being responsible, even for themselves. The middle of the line brings success in leadership and being responsible for others. And, as with all the lines, these abilities decline towards the end.

The second column represents the beginning of the process in taking responsibility for one's own person. A curious dream or delusion of the remedy Baryta carbonica is that they walk on their knees. This expresses the feeling of inability to stand up on their own – their inner structure is not sturdy enough to carry themselves, so they need help.

Amanda shows qualities that correspond to the core sensation of this remedy: she is extremely sensitive to being called a baby or having others think she behaves like a baby. We see this in several examples. She cannot handle responsibilities and learning materials that are hard for her. She cannot accomplish reading assignments without her mother's help. She is dependent on her. On the other hand we see how much she would love to be an independent thinker. She would like to be an adult and have her own credit card and pay her taxes. That is what, in her mind, makes an adult. This is a strong need in her, and that's why math is the subject that she is the most anxious about.

When her mother tells me that Amanda was developing normally during the first year of her life and then "fell apart," this is a hint of the frailty of Amanda's structure: she has built up some structure but it is very fragile. This is characteristic of the second column: there is a beginning structure but if challenged by the slightest stress, the person needs support. Just as Amanda's mother tells me, she can tackle very simple tasks or read easy material, but if it is even a little bit harder she needs her mom's support. If she needed a remedy from the first column she would have no "structure" whatsoever; she would be completely dependent on her mother. But that is not the case. She is capable of simple tasks.

When asking Amanda about her goals and main anxieties we come to the sensation of her not functioning properly in order to execute complex tasks; she would like to be an adult and live a responsible life. The stage she is at in the process of achieving this is in the beginning of development, just one step beyond the complete dependence on others' support. The first remedy Amanda receives is Baryta carbonica, in 200c potency.

Six weeks later, at the follow-up visit, Amanda's mom tells me that the only difference she has noticed is that a required book they were reading for school went much easier than she expected. Other than that Amanda has been tired and lethargic. At this point I recommend using a different potency of the same remedy, thinking that the first one started the healing process but was not the appropriate strength.

A few days later I get an email from Amanda's mom, telling me that she has had mononucleosis:

Hi Ildiko,
Amanda collapsed on Saturday, and we took her to the hospital. She has mono, unfortunately. Now she is recovering. She must have been sick for a while before she collapsed, so she seems to be at the end of mono rather than the beginning. I would like to give it a couple of weeks until she completely recovers before giving her any medication or remedy. I am not putting her back on Concerta® until she gets better.

> I tell her that homeopathy can offer help in speeding along the recovery from illnesses like mono, so even if she did not want to continue treatment for the sake of Amanda's mental development we could meet to evaluate her physical state. She decides she wants to wait with any kind of treatment, so I do not see them until four months later:

– *How has she been since taking the remedy?*
– Her attention is much better. She takes beautiful notes and pays attention. Last year she was spacing out more. Now her notes are good. She understands instructions. Last year it was very inconsistent; she struggled more. She took all the notes; she knew what she needed to know. To answer "why" and "how" are hard. She manages the "what," "who," and "when," But when

I ask "why" she tenses up right away and says. "I don't know." She gives up right away. If it requires thinking skills she will not even try. If I give her a little hint she can do it.

— *Say more about this inability to answer the "why" questions*

— She is afraid to say the wrong thing, rather does not say anything. Abstraction and analysis are hard for her. She won't even think. She knows it is hard for her, so she does not even try. If you break it down to simpler questions she will be able to do that.

— *What else have you noticed since the remedy?*

— She has become very interested in people; she seems to understand people more. She reads the book *Friendship Troubles*. At Halloween she managed to call her friend after she blew her off and went to another party without calling Amanda. So I told her she could call her and tell her how she felt. After this I saw her reading the book. Of course when I went by her room she quickly hid it. But then she called her and the girl was ice to her for two weeks. So it worked. This was a first experience for Amanda.

— *What kinds of things has she been talking about recently? What seems to be on her mind?*

— First and most importantly she talks about friends and friendships. If you ask about friends, she would say everything was okay. But she does not have close friends.

— *What about school?*

— She needs help with academics. She admits that she needs help to me and to her teachers, but the thing she cannot handle is if she is singled out – if the aid comes only to her and not to the others. She feels then, that the other kids see that she needs help. She is afraid that if she fails the test, she would stay behind. She has a hard time accepting any kind of help because she does not want anybody to know that she has a problem. She is covering it up. She is very sensitive to be singled out. She would have a meltdown if the aid came only to her. If she is treated differently, she feels everybody is gonna know! Her two main concerns are to be singled out, and what if others see her.

— *What about carrying on a conversation?*

– I have seen her on a roll with a conversation but usually just one-word answers. She is unsure what she understands. I think it is a fear of failure, like "I am afraid I am gonna get it wrong." She is afraid to say anything because someone is gonna make fun of her. She is still very sensitive to criticism.

Amanda comes in separately again.

– *Why didn't you want your mom to be here?*
– It's embarrassing.
– *Embarrassing?*
– Because you have done something and it is embarrassing.
– *Done what?*
– Nothing.

> She says this quickly as usual.
> This visit uncovers a few key elements that provide me with further details and enable me to pick a more suitable remedy. As I mentioned earlier, there are several salts of each mineral. With the Baryta group of remedies there are eleven homeopathic remedies made of various salts of Barium: Baryta carbonica, Baryta sulphurica, Baryta arsenica, Baryta iodata, Baryta phosphorica, etc. There are certain differences between these remedies that are not always easy to discern. In Amanda's case I started with Baryta carbonica and followed with Baryta sulphurica, which proved to be the one that helped her more profoundly. In situations like this, what happens is that some improvements are achieved by taking the first remedy but some essential issues remain untouched. A fine-tuned second prescription clears up the rest of the problem. We see the need for a different salt of the remedy when we can distinguish two parallel issues running in the core of the case. The problem cannot be summarized as a clear, single-focused issue. During this second visit I recognize the two parallel issues within Amanda's

sensation. It is not purely that she is not able to have responsibility, in which case Baryta carbonica, the single remedy, would be perfect for her.

But there is another consideration here. I still believe that Baryta is a part of her sensation. The question could arise whether she needs a remedy from the second column on a line above. In Amanda's sensation there is a definite amount of personal weight. As discussed in the first chapter, as we go lower in the periodic table, the weight of the personality increases, just as the atomic weight of the elements. In Amanda's case the strong sense of self can be seen in her emphasis on the fear of criticism and that others would laugh at her. If she had no strong sense of self she would not be ashamed or would not care about others talking about her. In that case she would need a remedy from one of the previous lines of the periodic table, one from the earlier stages of development. But Amanda's issues lie on the sixth line. She wants to live a responsible adult life, and she is capable of doing things. The fact that she needs help, like the little push her mother tells me about, and that she cannot handle complex questions but that once you start her off she can do it prove that her remedy is at the beginning of the line. Baryta seems appropriate.

The other half, the part that does not fit the Baryta carbonica picture, is related to Amanda's pride. Her ego surfaces, which points to another remedy: Sulphur. Her fear of failure is a typical fear of the sixth line, as these people have reached a high level – if they fall, they fall big. This, combined with the fear of others making fun of her, brings the salt Baryta sulphurica to mind: She is proud of who she is so she cannot bear to be criticized and fears failing or having made a mistake. Sulphur, as a single element, is proud of his identity, having reached the development of ego (being towards the end of the third line of the periodic table) where he has established himself as a separate identity from others. The remedy Baryta sulphurica blends the qualities of dependence and dignity. This best reflects the forces that are the core of Amanda's sensation.

A month later, Amanda's mom comes back and tells me:

– Soon after she took the remedy she got better. She has improved academically. She has had good reactions, good conversations. My sister, who spends quite a bit of time with her, commented on it. An incident happened the day after she took the remedy: Amanda was crying about an old friend, a girl who did not invite Amanda this year to her birthday party (while the previous years she did). As she was crying, she took her phone and erased the girl's number from her phone memory. This kind of social awareness is completely new. She used to deny all these issues. Later we had a great discussion about it, and she talked with my sister, too. She has also picked up the phone and called some friends without me initiating it.

In school she has a new aid, who was surprised to hear that I thought Amanda had social problems. She said Amanda hung out with other kids. This was not the case last year. Last week they had a test, and she wrote a one-and-a-half-page essay on her own! It is still hard for her to analyze situations, but with more factual information she is getting better and better. She is happier and less anxious! Her program consultant told me that she has a smile on her face now and seems to be happy in class. She asked me: "What have you done to her?"

She also eats more now. She still has trouble concentrating on her homework. She gets frustrated and says she cannot do it on her own – just sits and stares at it. She is better with retaining information, at least now she knows what to do for homework.

– *What about sensitivity to criticism?*

– She is a little less sensitive to criticism. She does not fly off the handle when someone has a sarcastic comment about her. She is better with conversation. That plateaued last week, I think.

At this point there is no need to repeat the remedy. Unless Amanda relapses, the remedy is still acting. A further dose would not speed up healing, and it might actually disturb the process.

Three months later I receive an email from Amanda's mother, summarizing Amanda's progress since taking the remedy fourth months earlier:

I wanted to share some changes in Amanda with you. I am getting informal reports from school that there is a positive shift in her academic performance: she is more together, and she is doing better. Her part-time aid emailed me that a number of Amanda's teachers remarked on how she has improved in the last few weeks. I also wanted to tell you about an incident we had on the weekend when I tried to help her with her math homework. She was taking her frustrations out on me and got mean, so I got very angry with her. She wrote me a beautiful letter of apology while I was out running errands later that day; it brought tears to my eyes. It was the first time that she was so articulate in a letter and in a conversation that followed. I haven't seen a difference in her social life but there is definite progress in other areas. I haven't given her any further doses of the remedy.

Amanda's case illustrates the importance of staying with a well-selected remedy as long as there is improvement, but once more detailed information gets revealed to be able to reevaluate and switch to a more accurately fitting one. This case also illustrates the importance of seeing the individual characteristics in the case. Amanda had many symptoms that are characteristic of autism: early fears, head banging, etc. These were not taken into as much consideration when searching for a remedy as the particular symptoms that not all autistic children have: sensitivity to criticism and not wanting others to think she was a baby. Following the specific, individual, and unique in a case leads us to the right remedy choice.

CHAPTER 3

A DEEPER UNDERSTANDING OF THE PLANT KINGDOM

One of the biggest breakthroughs that Dr. Sankaran achieved while developing the Sensation Method was his understanding of the plant kingdom. He realized that the survival technique of plants is their ability to adapt to environmental changes. Their sensitivity is the key issue in this process. He also realized that, just as with the mineral kingdom where we have the periodic table to categorize the minerals, so too do we have plant families into which we divide the plant species. When he started studying the homeopathic characteristics of plant remedies, he found that, indeed, there were common sensations among remedies that came from the same botanical families. He realized that these remedies can be grouped into these plant families and, just as minerals can be placed at the meeting points of rows and columns of the periodic table, plant remedies can be grouped within the plant family according to the miasm the remedy belongs to.

MIASMS

Miasm is a unique grouping of homeopathy, which I mentioned briefly in Chapter 1. The term was first used by Samuel Hahnemann, the founder of homeopathy. He realized that some of his patients were getting better for awhile but then relapsed. This was the recurring pattern: he would repeat the remedy, improvement would last for a certain time and then the person would relapse again. His patients did not achieve that perfectly healthy state he set as the goal of healing. Being an avid scholar and researcher he looked closely at this phenomenon. He studied the background of these people and discovered that those who had ancestors with similar chronic diseases shared some personality characteristics. They did not have the actual disease itself but had other physical, mental or emotional traits that he could trace back to the inherited energetic blueprint of the disease from previous generations. At his time these major diseases were mainly syphilis, gonorrhea and psoriasis. Later, other homeopaths included other diseases, namely tuberculosis and cancer. Dr. Sankaran added a few more, such as typhoid, malaria or leprosy. These groupings carry the name of the disease and mainly refer to a certain pattern of disease, which the disease itself manifests. For example, the characteristics of malaria cover cases of intermittent acute attacks of the disease. Between periodic attacks, the person experiences relative calmness. If one experiences any other illness in this fashion, a homeopath would call for the remedy belonging to the malaria kingdom. Thus, the name suggests an illness but most likely the person has nothing to do with the actual illness itself; it is just the degree and characteristic pattern of his or her illness.

When we are discussing plant remedies we differentiate between vital sensations. In one plant family all individual species will share the same sensation. What is different is the degree to which they experience that sensation.

A CASE OF MIGRAINES
AND MENSTRUAL CRAMPS

Daphne comes to see me after I had treated three people in her family. The interview flies by. She is open to my questions and talks very descriptively. Her physical complaints are migraines, some other recurrent headaches and debilitating menstrual cramps. She tells me:

– I have had headaches my whole life. Recently I have improved my lifestyle, removed stress factors, but I am still carrying these headaches with me. I also have chronic pain along the right side of my body. I have had that since I was backpacking through Europe twelve years ago. Sometimes it gets so bad that I cannot walk. It acts up when I do not get enough sleep.

I ask her to describe the physical sensation a little more.

– It feels as if the thighbone went too deep inside the hip socket so the right leg feels shorter than the left. This sensation makes me want to pull it out. As if there were not enough space in the hip.

She puts an emphasis on this sensation by gesturing with her hand as if she were pulling two things apart.

It is a distinct sensation so I probe into it deeper.

– I feel there should be more space, more air. The pain starts in my back and it goes down the leg… I had my first migraine when I was ten years old. It runs in my family: my mom had it, my sister has it and my niece does, too. The first time it came in the middle of the night. I tried to press on the eye, but it did not help. My sister had a genius idea to give me a pill for it. She sneaked the pill out of Mom's medicine cabinet. It did not help. In fact, nothing helped. It was an awful pain.

– What did you do in response to the pain?

– True to my nature, I did not want to wake up my parents. All through my childhood I tried to parent myself.

> Earlier in the interview she would go off on tangents in her descriptions. This time, I ask her to stay with the physical sensations of the headache. Useful information can be revealed by telling about one's childhood and intellectual understanding of their own story, but to find the shortest way to the correct remedy we usually need to concentrate on the sensation in the chief complaints. Describing deeper and deeper the most disturbing ailments, we can get more core information than covering many areas superficially.

– When I was in motion the pain lessened a little, so I remember pacing the room all night long in the dark because any noise or light would disturb me. Sometimes I got so desperate I thought the best solution would be to stick a knife in the eye where the pain was.

I have four brothers and a sister. The boys were much older so I was growing up only with my sister in the house. She was two years older than me and had a very intense personality. She had anger outbursts; she was a high maintenance person. That is why I did not want to cause problems for our parents. I was a low-key, good girl. I felt that our parents did not have the emotional capacity to care for me. I feared my father, and I never complained. Mom was 38, Dad 48 when they had me. As they were getting older I had to take care of them. They still need my care today. My father is 80. My mom died three and a half years ago. I was very close to her. It was hard for me to leave her and come to the U.S. I love my mom a lot. I always got unconditional love from her. I still feel it, even when she is dead.

> We go back to the headaches for further exploration.

– I get the migraines at least once a month before my period. The other kind of headache is stress related; that could come any time. Stress builds up in me. I wish I could let things flow. I feel the stress energetically, feel it building up. Then, eventually, I get a headache. My big issue is that I want to be in control. It is hard for me to let the universe take control. It is hard to trust what I am not in control of. Anxiety comes when I repeatedly try to control events. I just keep saying things, giving advice to people. If I cannot take action to take control at least I can say something. Instead of trusting I keep saying, keep repeating.

When I have the headache I feel like a little girl: helpless and wanting to be in the dark. Light irritates me. I try to relax my eye. It is the right eye I get this pain in. The dark is very soothing. I get nauseous, too.

– *What do you do to relieve the pain?*

– I press on it. I find pressure is helpful. I studied shiatsu so I use it on myself when I am in pain. In shiatsu we believe that pain is caused by energy imbalance. There is excess energy in some parts of the body and deficiency at another. I, for example, have excess gallbladder energy and deficient long-intestine energy. The idea is that the energy is flowing along the meridians and at certain places blockages occur. The pain arises because of the blockage. After pressing on these points of blockage, my system eventually releases. My breath releases, I feel I am letting go. I also have to go to the bathroom then.

I ask her to tell me more about the physical sensation.

– I feel tightness in the muscles of the back. It is tight and there is pressure. It is like a rope that tightens up. There is no energy there. Along with this I have weakness in the lower back.

I ask her to describe it. I note that she has mentioned the word "flow" several times. When someone uses a phrase or word repeatedly, it places emphasis on it. Once we arrive at it from different complaints and perspectives, we know this is the core sensation.

At this point of the interview, while describing this flow, she uses another sensation-describing word: tight. So I inquire further: either she will describe the tightness as flow or the flow as tightness. There is always one core sensation to which all other sensations boil down to. In plant remedies this core sensation is experienced along with its opposite pair. Daphne mentions the sensation "flow" with its opposite of having blocks in the way. If she comes to the sensation "tight" as the underlying sensation, she will describe its opposite as well. Let's see what she says.

– It is like when you have a tight muscle.
– *Describe this more.*
– It is condense in place. There is no space to breathe, to relax. It is blocked. The whole system is blocked. There is no flow inside.

> So it is not the tightness but the block to the flow that is the sensation! Interesting to note how she describes the "no space" in the tight muscle and rope. It is very similar to the way she describes her complaint in the right side of the body and the hip socket. This means that in two areas of the body she feels a similar sensation, which makes the local sensation a general one and thus confirms its importance.
>
> I ask her to say more about the flow. If she keeps describing the flow and its opposite, the blocks, we know we are at the core sensation. If she leaves the flow behind and describes a different sensation, we will have to follow that to see what is at the core.

– I am aware of energy flow. Generally, there is flow in my body. When I am in pain everything gets stuck in my upper back, neck and head. The rest of the body is weak because the energy is stuck.
– *What is the opposite of this stuck energy and weakness?*
– When everything flows. I get an image of channels, meridians. When there is no block the breath flows, movement flows. It is a peaceful feeling, a sense of balance. There is energy available to walk, play and work. When I am in pain it feels as if someone put some stuff in my head that should not be there. It feels as if

it is going to explode if you keep stuffing it. The container of the head is too small. There is no space in it.

– No space?

– I have an image of the head with bubbles popping up in it. Just pressing them back does not help. Things will pop up again, somewhere else. All the energy goes up towards the head. It helps to ground myself. A hot bath can bring all that energy down. Once it goes up it gets stuck in the head.

– Describe this going up and down.

– It is flowing. It is fast. This energy is fast like a brook. Not like a river; it is faster than that. It can flow fast because there are no blocks in it. If I press on my feet it removes the blocks. In a similar fashion if I put my lower back in hot water the energy can flow back down. I have weakness in my back. I wish I had more energy flow. When I have a headache the head empties itself out of energy. That is what improves with hot water. It is relaxing. I can breathe. It is calling the energy down. It retracts the energy back, sucks it back. A slow, soft process of sucking it back.

> Even though these processes occur in our body, we usually are not aware of them and do not discuss them during everyday conversation. In the homeopathic interview these sensations unfold in a graceful manner, and even though some people are taken back by the "nonsense" they are describing, it is often eye-opening to point out these inner sensations that feed our body awareness and our view of reality. Once the person feels it is a safe environment to talk about these processes, they are more open to discussing them and are not surprised by my interest of details regarding the nature of this inner reality.

– What do you mean by calling the energy down?

– It is a soft bubbling. In the large intestine meridian I sense popping, bubbling and releasing. The energy that was stuck up in the head finally releases. Empty places start to fill up. As a result there is less pressure in the head. It cannot pop up anymore.

I picture the body as a vessel. There is a certain amount of energy or liquid it can contain. In imbalance there is too much in one area, another area is empty. When there is balance it evens out.

> This image is clear and specific and contains other sensations that Daphne describes before all boil down to the sensation of flow. Therefore, at this point we can move on to another area and bring that down to the same sensation. I ask her to describe her menstrual cramps.

– I have always thought everyone had cramps; it was so natural for me. It is awful, so much pain. I lie in bed in pain. I would put a hot water bottle on my belly and take Ibuprofen©. It is a nightmare. I cannot function; I have no energy. The feeling is that something is shrinking inside. It is tight and then it releases. It contracts. Every time it contracts it hurts.
– *Please tell me about your hobbies.*

> We ask about hobbies because the energy of the vital sensation manifests clearly through them. People seek the opposite of their core sensation, which they create in their hobbies. It is the same energy manifesting in two polarities. If a person experiences pain with a sensation they usually seek the opposite in their work, leisure activities, dream-vacation, favorite movies and books. It is not only useful for us to see what the opposite of the core sensation is, it also brings a pleasant energy to the interviewing process as the person can describe and re-experience something they truly enjoy.

– I like playing basketball and hiking, and I love reading. I have done different kinds of martial arts. My favorite is contact improvisation dance. It is about sharing your weight with a partner and flowing with it. It creates balance. I work as a movement therapist. The aspect of it I enjoy the most is that people connect with each other. I love moving myself. I feel the body opens and there is more connection. I am very much a

moving person. I love running, dancing – I love any movement.
I put all my heart into it. I like action and flow: movement,
momentum, motion. When I throw a basketball I put my whole
body in it.
– *How do you feel when you are in motion?*
– Happy!

   She giggles.

– I feel pleasure; I am high. I even have dreams about it. I walk
in my dream and then go into a flight-motion. I rise up while
walking. My whole body is happy. It is a physical and emotional
sensation. I feel power, flow, radiance and fun. It is a child-like
feeling. At times I laugh out loud. There is a surprise piece in it,
which I like. I do not know what is going to happen. There is no
structure; it is all improvisation. Anything can happen when I
manage to flow with it. I feel soft, flexible and strong at the
same time.

   I ask her to describe how it feels like to be soft, flexible
   and strong.

– Like a rubber doll. I feel like I can do anything. There is no
stiffness. Everything flows. It is like a waterfall, like a river.

   This image brings together the quality and depth of
   Daphne's core sensation. She experiences pain and
   weakness as blocked flow. She is working on
   reestablishing the flow whenever she has headaches or
   cramps. She either presses points known to release
   those blocks or she sits in a hot bath to reestablish the
   flow of energy in her body. She mentions three areas
   in her life where she enjoys the sensation of flow: her
   work, shiatsu and contact improvisation dance. The
   way she describes these activities is essentially the same:
   they create flow and ease of movement. This is the
   opposite of the blocked sensation. This is the sensation-
   pair that we see in the plant family Daphne's remedy
   comes from. To find the exact remedy within the family,
   we use the depth of her sensation of flow and blockage.

This depth is her desire to control overwhelming situations. She talks about struggling, of letting go of control. On the other hand, in contact improvisation dance she enjoys the improvisational aspect of the movement and likes the unpredictability, how she does not need to control it: she can let go, flow freely. These two aspects together define her remedy, Thlaspi, that comes from the plant Shepherd's purse.

Daphne takes the remedy in 200c potency and comes back for a visit four weeks later. She reports:

– I feel it really worked. The cramps were less painful. At some point I took Ibuprofen® but only once! Usually I take it every hour. Usually my period is a nightmare; now it was less intense. The headaches are tricky to evaluate. I had some tension in my back. I tried to let it flow and in fact it did not turn into a massive headache. Once I was sad and I could not cry about it. It was a heavy sadness. I felt blocked. If I had cried it would not have turned into a headache. I wish I could cry. I did cry after the remedy! I was on the phone with a friend, I cried and the headache did not develop at all. I was surprised that I cried. I feel the remedy opened something. I have less resistance in a lot of areas.

– *What do you mean by less resistance?*

– I mean less resistance to look at things. For example, as I told you I am trying to save everybody. On one hand it is a good skill but on the other hand I compromise my needs. Since taking the remedy, I feel many possibilities have opened up. I have been able to think about myself in simple things, like when someone asks me if I want tea or coffee. I am not used to thinking in terms of *my* needs.

Also, at work I noticed I was more focused on my task. Normally it would disturb me when people are talking in the same room where I am sitting. I would listen to them and try to help... now I focus on my work. The headaches are less in general, less intense. I am able to let go. If not, then it turns into a bad headache.

During follow-up visits like this one, I am looking for several things. One is improvement regarding the person's complaints. In Daphne's case, these are her headaches, cramps and backache. She reports improvement in all those areas. Another improvement we are looking for is that of the sensation. This is something that the person is not consciously aware of. Even though all the sensations boil down to this core sensation, people usually do not come to see a homeopath complaining about the core sensation. This is something that the homeopath elicits from the interview. At the follow-up visits we are most eagerly looking for changes in this core sensation.

Once we touch the core sensation we know healing is under way. The core sensation is the closest expression of the human body to the core imbalance that we are addressing. Everything else is nothing but mere manifestation of this core. Hence, even though the person is getting relief while the complaints are going away, the real cure comes when the sensation melts away. If the person experiences even a small portion of the original complaints, if they describe the sensation the same way, we know healing is not yet complete. Sometimes the actual complaint is not gone but while talking about it the person is obviously relieved of the sensation. That is a sign of increasing health.

At this follow-up visit, Daphne provides hints that her healing happened in terms of the flow, which is her core sensation. Even though I first concluded the core sensation without her realizing what it was, by now she has developed an understanding of it and realizes that when the flow was established she felt better. Becoming aware is the beginning of healing. So Daphne's first reaction to the remedy is promising.

At this point I tell her to repeat the remedy Thlaspi in case the cramps or headaches came back with her next period. She started off on a good healing path but her headaches kept coming back and her period still caused pain. I do not repeat the remedy automatically at the time of the visit as she has no complaints, but the recurrent quality of the complaints implies that they might come back at their regular time. If they do, that is a good time to repeat.

Four months later Daphne sends me an email. She tells me that her symptoms keep improving but along the way she experiences some related issues.

I am doing better with my symptoms. I rarely have headaches and when I do they are not as strong. The menstrual cramps are still there. I will try to notice if there is change in the intensity when I get my period again. What I struggle with now is anxiety. I will write to you after my period, which should be coming up any day. Thanks again, Daphne.

At the next follow-up visit it will become clear that the anxiety coexists with a physical symptom, shortness of breath, that she had experienced earlier in her life. In this email Daphne does not mention the shortness of breath, as she does not think it is related to her homeopathic treatment. Only in talking to her do I find out about her medication that she used for her shortness of breath, and in turn she got back the physical symptom that came up as a result of anxiety in the past. This is a good example of how suppressing physical symptoms can manifest on the emotional and mental levels. Without having all the puzzle pieces we cannot solve these mysteries. In this case I could not understand why the anxiety came up as the headaches were getting better. The natural pattern of the disease leaving the body is that the more important layers heal first. The emotional layer is more important (i. e., deeper seated) than the physical. That is why usually the emotional layer heals first and physical symptoms might linger longer. It should not happen the other way around. Once we understand that Daphne experienced a return of old symptoms (a part of the healing journey) and that it was suppressed with the inhaler, the events make sense for us as homeopaths. She experienced anxiety, an emotion that manifested in the past as the same physical ailment: shortness of breath. As you will see in the recount of the following visits, Daphne's homeopathic treatment clears up the physical complaint and the anxiety behind it, and her headaches and menstrual cramps further improve.

She comes in a couple of weeks later:

– It is not only the anxiety I feel more prominently now; I also have shortness of breath. Two months ago I got a bad cold, then it went away but a dry cough stayed. I coughed all the time. I went to the doctor who gave me two inhalers, one with Albuterol® and another with a steroid. I used it for one week and the cough was improving a lot. Then it came back. Ever since I have been using the inhaler daily. It seems to relieve the symptoms but does not get rid of the problem. Inhaling is fine, but when I would exhale it gets constricted and then it comes up to the throat and I cough. I feel the air path contracting, shrinking and sometimes getting stuck. I had the same symptoms many years ago and then they gave me an inhaler, too. I know stress brings it out. Back then the source of the stress was that I had a person who moved in with me and I could not ask her to move out. My usual problem surfaced again: putting other people's needs in front of mine. I was considering whether to move out myself but was too scared to do that either. I thought I would hurt her feelings. I was scared of her reaction, that she would be mad at me. I think it is the same reaction as the one I had to my father. I felt unloved. He punished me by not talking to me, and so I wanted to please him. I felt scared for not having the control over when he would be angry. I felt very alone when he would not talk to me. I felt unprotected, not cared for. So that is how I tried to be really good. I was an A student and behaved well.

> Here Daphne is talking about the physical complaint and the accompanying anxiety, which could have been unrelated unless explained in the context of her history. In fact, both the anxiety and the breathing problem are old weak spots in her that have now resurfaced. This is a good example of homeopathy's holistic nature. Treatment includes all facets of the person's health. All symptoms are part of the whole – our job is to see where they fit it. In this case shortness of breath was a returning old symptom, which had to come to the surface as it was suppressed with medication in the past. Homeopathic treatment is like a spring-cleaning: it brings out all the debris from the body, exposes them and offers them for us to clean out. With the right non-suppressive treatment, these issues can be dealt with and cleared out for good.

– My periods are much better, though the first day I still have pain. I had a headache two weeks ago. I have not had it so bad for years! The intensity was so strong. I was throwing up; it lasted the whole day. The day before I had a Contact Improvisation session where we did an authentic movement. I worked with closed eyes for ten minutes.

> I ask her to tell me about the experience she had during that movement.

– It was a process. In the beginning I felt very young, like a baby. Then I experienced hesitating movements, then growing up, more expressive movements. I feared something might stop the movement from expressing itself. It was a fear of taking up too much space. A fear of my own power, a fear of the flow. My movements got jerky, not flowing. But it felt very real. It was a fear of being full, big and expressive. I felt a block that stops.
– *What is that block?*

– Putting other people's needs first. The block was inside the movement. The movement was choppy. The nature of movement is that it has blocks.

– *Choppy?*

– Uncomfortable.

> This description is another confirmation of her innermost sensation, the flow and the blocks in it. There have been improvements in her health and in her sense of flow, but the fact that she is still describing this sensation hints that her healing is not yet complete. Describing this dip in her improvement illustrates again how everything in the body and mind is related: she starts improving while on the homeopathic remedy, which brings the old problem to the surface. Not only does it stay with her, bringing anxiety along, but she also experiences an aggravation in her migraines as well as her energetic expression during contact improvisation dancing, where her usual sense of flow becomes "choppy and blocked."
>
> I ask about the pain in her back and hip and she tells me that she has not had any pain in the hip. The weakness in the right side has reduced as well. I recommend that she take the remedy "as needed." I tell her that every time she feels the need for the inhaler she could instead try a dose of the remedy in 30c potency. This potency is more capable of helping with acute physical problems or ones that are somatic manifestations of emotional problems, like her anxiety in this situation.
>
> A month later, she reports:

– Since I took the remedy, I stopped using the inhaler. I got a cold and was feeling pretty sick but then I got better. I have been having headaches and tension in my body. I miss the sense of flow I have had since we started treatment. I have so much tension all over.

At this point I give Daphne the same remedy in 200c potency. The next email comes three months later:

My headaches and cramps are better. I still have headaches once in a while, especially before my period, but I have less. The cramps are definitely less intense than they used to be. The breath problems I had were gone within a few days! You are a genius. Now every time someone has breathing issues and is prescribed an inhaler, I tell them to talk to you instead. Thank you again, for everything.

Notice how I had determined that Daphne again needed the original potency. The 30c helped her to overcome the physical ailment but was unable to reestablish the flow, which the original 200c potency was able to start healing. Theoretically, I might be wondering what would have happened if she had not turned to conventional medicine when she had the shortness of breath but had consulted me instead. That return of her old symptom was a sign of healing and could have been addressed with homeopathy. Instead, we have to make this loop of getting her back in track and deal again with our ultimate goal: achieving the sensation of flow and removing the blocks.

After another three months go by, Daphne comes back for a follow-up visit. Even though her cramps and headaches were gone for a while, she suddenly experienced her old backache. As we discuss what has happened she tells me she had a stressful time and drank some coffee for a few days. That is when the backache came back. It seems most likely that she antidoted the remedy with the coffee.

Coffee is one of the substances that have been noted for their effects to negate a remedy's action. Some homeopaths warn their patients not to drink coffee at all while under homeopathic treatment. Yet it seems that people who regularly drink coffee and are not affected by it will not have problems with it while taking the remedy. People who are not coffee drinkers might drink an occasional cup and it really gives them a huge boost.

These situations might affect their healing progress if it is in close proximity to the time they took a homeopathic remedy.

The latest report I have from Daphne is that all her symptoms are improving. The remaining symptom is some occasional menstrual cramps. She took a dose of her remedy in 10M potency. This accelerated her healing a great deal. The 10M might have been the potency she needed in the first place. Potency is selected according to the level the person is experiencing their complaints at. When someone talks about the core sensation with ease, like Daphne, the right potency is often 10M. However, sometimes there are some considerations that point to a lower potency initially. This is what happened in this case.

Daphne's case illustrates some of the challenges in long-term case management. Homeopathic remedies are deep acting and bring on long-lasting healing. Nevertheless, there are always ups and downs, different stresses in people's lives that can bring back old symptoms. Some symptoms might go and return for awhile. In some cases, some symptoms are suppressed, so we have to make sure healing continues by solving these problems. In any case, the well-placed placed homeopathic remedy in the right dose can help people through crises and guide them towards further healing. Sometimes the best strategy is to wait, sometimes it's a new remedy and sometimes it's the same remedy in a different potency. The right response always depends on our understanding of the case in depth. We have to know the history of the person, the quality and duration of complaints. These are fine differences and it always depends on the core sensation. That is the compass in telling the homeopath what is the right decision at the moment.

Some people are surprised when they describe their current symptoms and receive the same remedy they were given for some other ailment. On the superficial level the new symptoms might not resemble the previous complaints. But as they talk about it, about the deeper core of the sensation, it often comes to the same inner sensation. Hence, the same remedy is needed. This usually happens later, when the person has experienced a long period of health.

In some instances, describing the new symptoms will reveal a different inner sensation. In that case a different remedy is needed. We cannot judge without looking at the depth of the actual sensation in the ailment.

In the following case, you will notice that the remedy is the same as Daphne's although the complaint is very different. The prescription is based solely on the symptoms of the acute situation, not on chronic or constitutional case-taking.

A Case of Acute Kidney Colic
A Case Taken By Anna Menyhért and Supervised by Ildiko Ran

I meet Sophie just after she was discharged from the hospital. She had gone there because of vomiting, great pain and fainting. She also could not pass urine. When she was admitted to the hospital she found out she had two kidney stones, one of which was in the kidney while the other one had moved down to the ureter, causing the excruciating pain. She was given painkillers, and her urine mixed with pus and blood was drained through a catheter. She was discharged from the hospital with the hope that she would spontaneously pass the stones during the weekend. That is when we meet. We talk for about twenty minutes, while a casual conversation turns into case taking session.

> I ask her how she is doing. In response, she tightens her two hands in fists and pulls them downward in front of her chest as she speaks.

– It is cramping and contracting.

> Since Sophie is in acute pain and feels miserable there is no need to approach her vital sensation carefully and gradually as I do with chronic ailments. By asking her as a well-meaning, interested sympathizer, I prompt her to describe her innermost experience, and gesturing with her hands confirms the significance of her expression. Looking at her talking and gesturing makes me think how easy it would be to find the right remedy for her. As a test I ask her what the opposite of this state would be.

– That would be releasing and relaxing. But now it is pulling down, tightens, and I need to relax in order for it to release.

> I ask her to show me with her hands how it is when she feels well. Spontaneously she opens her fists in front of her belly.

– I feel fine for a while, and then it starts again. It cramps where the stone is.

> She pulls her fists in again.

– Then it smoothes out.

> She gestures with open palms.

– It bounces back to normal. Then the cramp eases; I become sleepy and tired. If I am not too tired I start walking up and down the stairs so the stone will come out.

– *Describe just the two hand gestures.*

– It tightens and hurts. Then releases and lets go. Clinging onto something, gripping, then letting go.

> Since she is talking about two distinct sensation opposites, I know she needs a plant remedy. I ask her whether these sensations are familiar to her.

– I often have similar sensations. Giving birth, having diarrhea, intestinal blocks. Tightens, cramps up, and then it releases. This cramp is similar to the contractions in labor. It feels as if I gave birth again.

> Since she is very tired and weary about going deeper into these sensations, I try from a different angle.

– *Do you have recurrent dreams?*

– Yes. I am with a large group of people, at familiar places, in a large building, like my old high school. Various things are happening at various locations and I am in all of those. We don't use stairs but slide on slides.

– *How is the feeling of sliding on slides?*

– Good. Quickly changing. I can be at different places at the same time. I am light, fast, sleek and self-confident.

– *If not?*

– That's not good. It evokes anxiety. Unpredictable, I do not know what is happening.

– *Please tell me more about that.*

– Uncertainty. Unstable feeling. The moment before fainting. It is related to the cramp. Eventually I don't faint and the moment before fainting lasts forever. I never know if the next moment I really faint or it stays as it is.

– What does it depend on whether or not you faint?

– I cannot control it. It is like a frozen moment.

– Cannot control it?

– I am not inside it. I am waiting, as an outsider, for what is going to happen.

– What does it feel like to be at different places at the same time?

– I am not left out from anything.

– And how does it feel to be left out?

– In that case I am an observer; I am not part of it. I am not there to know about things.

– How is the sliding on slides?

– Change of location. Fast, funny, no blocks, smooth.

– And if there are blocks?

– Those need to be eliminated in a fast, smart and effective way.

> At this point Sophie tells me she is tired and nervous. She asks to stop the conversation, as she is not prepared to talk about these sensations. As a last question I ask her what she is afraid of.

– I am afraid of the cramps, that I would get into that state before fainting. Because I don't know what to do with it. In that state, things are happening to me; I have no way to have a say. I have no control over what happens to me.

At this time she does not want to take any homeopathic remedies, so I have a chance to think over what she has told me. It happens to people when they seek advice from an acquaintance, who happens to be a homeopath, that at the end they hesitate to take the remedy. Since I have heard about this natural tendency of people I am not truly surprised by her reluctance to take the remedy, but I want to be ready as soon as she wants to try it.

She returns to the hospital where they attempt – with no success – to break up the stones with laser. She calls me from the hospital saying her next option is surgery, which she would like to avoid. She asks for the homeopathic remedy.

Here's how I evaluate Sophie's situation: The diseased state – the cramp – shows itself as a block, a frozen moment, whereas the healthy state is a smooth flow with no blocks. This sensation pair is recurrent in Sophie's history and the positive side comes across in her dream as well. In the Sensation Method this pair are attributes of the plant family Cruciferae.

The most disturbing aspect for Sophie is her inability to affect and control her situation. This points to the miasm her remedy belongs to. The characteristic of this miasm is that the person is trying to cope with a situation that is well beyond her capabilities. Among the members of the plant family Cruciferae it is Thlaspi, the remedy made of the plant Shepherd's Purse, that reflects this miasm. Among the key symptoms of Thlaspi we find kidney stones, painful urination, spasmodic retention of urine, kidney colic, urethritis and urine mixed with blood and pus.

One of the important characteristics of Thlaspi is a desire or impulse to walk and pace. As we see in Sophie's case, whenever she is not too tired she walks up and down with the hope of passing the stones. We saw this same symptom in Daphne's case as well where she was also pacing up and down while having a migraine. In the Sensation Method we rely on the repertory, just as in any branch of homeopathy, even though these are mainly used for confirmation here. In other methods of classical homeopathy, mental and general symptoms are the most significant. We can imagine many different reactions to headaches or kidney colic, but the fact that Daphne and Sophie both reacted with pacing and walking up and down is certainly significant.

While we wait for the remedy to arrive, I suggest that Sophie draw a doodle because sometimes just looking at the doodle often brings about a healing effect. So while in the hospital Sophie draws a doodle on a napkin. Then she looks at it and writes down the words that come to her mind. In about an hour she feels a little sharp pain and subsequently passes one of the stones.

The doctors tell her that in case the other stone does not move they will do the surgery the following week.

Sophie goes home again. Because she fells a little more energized than she had the previous week, I decide on a relatively high potency diluted in water. I tell her to sip the water a few times within the next couple of hours until she starts feeling better. After taking one sip of the diluted remedy, she calms down completely and falls asleep.

The next morning she feels strong. She develops a skin rash but it does not bother her. Then, the next day she feels worse again. She is disappointed, afraid that passing the stone will be painful. She also complains about her period that had started a few days earlier and then froze. I recommend that she drink again from the remedy, especially because the expression "frozen" implies the sensation she talked about earlier. The next morning she passes the second stone without pain. She has avoided surgery.

This case is an illustration of acute situations when we can quickly reach the vital sensation and find a curative remedy without probing into the chronic issues of the client. In Chapter 4 you will read about a case where the curative remedy for an acute condition was found through the client's chronic picture, hence proving that her acute situation was in fact a part of her general makeup.

A CASE OF RECURRENT HEAD LICE

A Case Taken By Anna Menyhért and Supervised by Ildiko Ran

Martha, a fourteen-year-old girl, has a problem with head lice. Through a pre-appointment conversation with her mother, I learn that Martha had first gotten head lice about six months ago and that she has not been able to get rid of them. Her mother also tells me that Martha has changed since becoming a teenager. Now everything seems boring to her. She has stopped playing sports and wants to dance instead, and she is not clear about her talents and skills. Also, everything is extreme with Martha – either black or white. Otherwise, she has no physical complaints. She rarely gets sick, and if she gets a cold she shakes it off easily. Other than the head lice, the only significant problem the mother sees is that ever since she was little, Martha has had trouble falling asleep. Martha comes in alone to talk to me.

– *What would you like help with?*

– The head lice are not going away, and half of my hair fell out and I have no idea why.

– *When did this start?*

– I don't know. All I noticed was that earlier my hair was thick and now it is not. Once I was brushing my hair and I realized there was nothing. That was bad.

– *There was nothing?*

– I had no hair.

– *You had no hair?*

– Of course I do have hair, but earlier when I would grab it there would be a lot of it and now, if I collect it in a ponytail, it is only a few hairs. And it is ugly.

– *How did you get the head lice?*

– My classmates and my best friend had it.

– *How did it happen? Did you just notice it one day?*

– I am not sure. I noticed I had no hair, not the lice. I told my mom it did not look good. She checked my head and then we saw them. Later the nurse came to our class and checked everybody and I still had it, even though by then we had got rid of them once. But they did not go away. Then we tried again and they did not leave that time either.

— *Tell me why this is bad. In what way does it bother you? How do you feel about it?*

— I am becoming uglier and uglier. This mushroom haircut is really outdated.

>   She used to have nice long hair, which they cut.

— *Because of the hairdo?*

— Yes, because I have so little hair now and the others have much more.

— *Others have more?*

— Yes, my best friend's hair is really beautiful.

— *How does that make you feel?*

— Sometimes I feel a little sad about my hair not being as nice, but I cannot do anything about it.

— *Tell me more about being sad about it.*

— That happens when I am bored. I think it is not fair that my friend has such nice hair. I am not envying her, not at all.

— *What happened when you touched your hair and felt there was nothing?*

— There were only a few hairs.

— *What was your feeling when that happened?*

— I got scared: where is my hair? I had not noticed until then that it had been falling out maybe for six months or even a year. All of a sudden I saw a lot of hair all over my room. That was scary. And when I would wash it, I could easily pull out a whole clump.

>   This is accompanied by a hand gesture: Martha is pulling and twisting a clump of hair and then suddenly yanks it.

— *Tell me exactly what you felt when you touched your hair, got scared, pulled out a clump while washing…*

— Oh, no… what can I do now?

— *How did that feel?*

– Really bad. I had no idea what to do. I thought everything would be all right soon – that my hair would quickly grow thick again if we just got rid of the lice. But it does not work. My hair keeps falling. When I was brushing it and ran my fingers through it, so much hair came out that I had to stop brushing.

– *What did you feel then?*

– That there was nothing I could do. I was helpless: "Oh, no!" I got nervous that we had treated it three times and it was not going away and I didn't know why. I felt miserable.

– *Why do you think it is not going away?*

– I keep getting it from different people. When I'm with my friend and we are writing or doing anything together, our heads are right next to each other. When I sleep over at her house, I sleep in her queen-size bed with her, and she always comments about how much hair I leave there.

– *How is your relationship with your friend? What do you do together?*

– We play. We make fun of everything, just cracking up. It is hard to describe – it is just a lot of fun to be with her.

– *Is there anything you have done together that especially stands out?*

– I have lots of fun memories, but when I talk about them, nobody understands – only the kids our age.

– *What does funny mean to you?*

– If someone says something amusing, or when someone makes fun of something serious.

– *What is that like? Why do you like to make fun of serious things?*

– Because it is hilarious. We are not crazy about serious stuff.

– *Why?*

– Because we get bored with it. Serious stuff is not fun; it is boring. It is much better to do something exciting.

– *Exciting? What is that like?*

– It makes me excited.

– *How is that? How does it affect you?*

– My heart is racing. I have to bounce up and down: now something needs to happen. I am so excited.

– *You have to bounce?*

– I am in high spirits. For instance, if I got a good grade on my

test, I have to yell out loud, "Woohoo! Cool! That's it, at last!"
That's the feeling.

> At this point of the session, I have a rough idea of
> what is going on with Martha. She has recurrent
> episodes of head lice, but what disturbs her the most
> is that her hair falls out and makes her feel ugly.
> Interestingly, she does not even notice the lice at first,
> only the excessive thinning of the hair. She thinks
> she might have had lice well before she discovered it.
> When she notices her hair is falling out, she fells two
> things: scared ("Oh, no!") and a sense of not knowing
> what to do.
>
> Head lice are parasites and thus can point to the malarial
> miasm, which is found at the meeting point of the
> acute and the sycotic miasms. The "Oh, no!" expresses
> the sensation of the acute miasm, featured by a sudden
> critical situation, while Martha's sense of not being able
> to do anything about it indicates the acceptance of the
> situation, which is a characteristic of the sycotic miasm.
> The acute and sycotic miasms together, or rather
> alternating with each other, lead to the malarial miasm,
> where, parallel to the characteristics of the illness,
> periods of inactivity alternate with acute flare-ups, a
> situation that the sufferer accepts as inevitable.

— *How is it that your friend's hair is more beautiful than yours?*
— She's just much more beautiful, very pretty.
— *And you?*
— I am not pretty because my hair is weird. And I am a little
chubby, too. Not always, only when I snack on candy bars at
night. In the middle of the night I go downstairs and get some.
— *Why do you do that?*
— Because I cannot sleep. And just for fun, for the heck of it.
— *How is it for you when you cannot sleep?*
— I stare at the stars, if the window is not hazy, and then I fall
asleep.

I note that several times Martha mentions her friend in relationship to her problem: she has beautiful hair, Martha sleeps at her house often, she plays with her, and they do funny things together. The significance of funny things catches my attention when she uses the same word in describing her inability to sleep: "just for fun." So fun or funny, which is related to exciting, is important for Martha in a general sense, not only in relation to her friend. When I ask her about the friend's beautiful hair, probing to determine whether or not she needs a remedy from the animal kingdom, she refers to funny again. At this point I start leaning towards a plant remedy for her: she keeps repeating the same sensation in different contexts and situations. From now on, I will be listening closely for any further references to "funny" or "exciting."

I am also noting that our conversation so far has been rather choppy. Martha has been answering all my questions very briefly. So I decide to ask her to tell me about a day in her life. I want her to talk freely and at length about something she feels comfortable with.

– I wake up in the morning; I am still sleepy. What am I supposed to say?

– *Whatever comes to your mind, just say it.*

– Okay. I eat breakfast, I dress up, I go to school, I enter the classroom, I say, "Hi, how are you?" The first period starts. Then recess, classes, recess. I eat lunch. Tuesday afternoon piano, Thursday English. The other days I go home, or at most I go to see my friend.

– *Do you like school?*

– Yes, I love it.

– *Why?*

– I like the atmosphere. The school is nice; it is amusing to be there.

I note that the only personal perspective she offers in

regards to school is about being amusing, which is very similar to fun and funny. So I ask about that.

– *You say amusing. Is amusement and fun important for you?*

– I don't even know what else could I come up with as a good thing.

– *Why?*

– When I am happy and amused I don't have to think about anything like my weird hair.

– *What about the time when you are not happy?*

– I don't talk.

– *You don't talk?*

– I am just sitting and there is nothing. Then nothing matters.

– *There is nothing?*

– I am not doing anything.

– *You are not doing anything?*

– I am moaning that, "Oh, I've had enough. I am bored." Or I start eating: I eat something yummy and then I feel better.

– *How is it when there is nothing?*

– I don't feel well, I am bored, I constantly want to eat because I have nothing to do.

– *And if you are happy?*

– Then I laugh and am able to say funny things.

– *How is it when you laugh and are able to say funny things?*

– Sometimes it is tiring for others, and me too, if we take it too far. Then there is no stopping us. We laugh so hard that we are rolling on the floor, holding our sides.

– *No stopping?*

– That is a great feeling: it is funny and stays with us for a long time. Afterwards we can ask each other: do you remember?

By now it is clear that Martha's case is about a pair of two opposites, which confirms the plant kingdom. The opposite of funny, happy, exciting is the boring, doing nothing, "there is nothing." Martha uses that last phrase related to her experience of seeing her hair falling out: "there is nothing." It seems as if this

"there is nothing" is not merely a local sensation but
a general one, running through the whole case.

– Funny, happy – this is important, right? On one hand, you have funny, happy and on the other hand, "there is nothing," you are bored. Is this right? Is there anything else?

– Only that it would be great to compete in something.

– Compete?

– To be a pro in something. Not because of the pride but because then I could tell the others: "Hey, do you know what happened, how great it was?"

– Why would it be good to be a pro in something?

– Because that is exciting.

– Exciting?

– Everybody thinks it is exciting to win something.

– How is it to win something?

– I never felt it. I have never won anything. But it must be: "Oh, this is great; I am so happy."

– How come you never won anything?

– At practices I was always last or the one before last.

– How did that feel?

– First it was terrible; I thought the world would come to an end. But next time I didn't care, so much so that I actually had fun.

– The world comes to an end?

– Oh, no, I am the last, it is so bad, everybody got to the next round, it must be so good for the winner: she succeeded in something and she has the skills. This must be a good point for her, a foothold, that she is good at it.

– Foothold?

– If you have a best friend, that is a foothold. You know about her that she loves you, and you love her.

> The issue of competition could lead to the sensation
> of the animal or mineral kingdom, if it were an issue
> of winner-loser or the performance-lack in structure.
> Instead, it is a tool for connection for Martha: if she

is a pro, skilled in something, she can tell her friends about it.

I also note that she refers again to excitement, this time as it comes from competing and winning. And from there, she refers again to the topic of friendship. The question now is whether making a connection is the ultimate goal for her or whether she would like to achieve something else by her connections. Considering the whole case, I conclude that she needs these connections so she can get out of the state of "nothing" to experience the funny-happy sensation. Now we will see further confirmations of this conclusion. For the time being I return to my previous question and leave the inquiry about the friend for later.

– *End of the world?*

– I will be sad: why didn't I succeed? It would have been so good.

– *And then what do you think?*

– Either that there will be something better or that nothing matters, that I cannot do anything about it; I am a dumbo; that's it.

The "cannot do anything about it" and the "that's it" return, indicating the acceptance of her limits according to the malarial miasm.

– *I am a dumbo?*

– Others are good and I am not.

– *Why is it important that others are good and you are not?*

– I don't envy them. It is okay if others are good but I want everybody to have some fun, even those who have less fun than those who have more fun. I don't think about myself but about everybody who has less fun than those who actually have fun. It is unfair that some have lots of fun and some not at all. But it is not the case that I don't have any fun at all. That is not true.

– *But?*

– I have fun in lots of things, but not in everything.

– *What could you do so you would have more fun?*

– I don't know.

Martha gets a little sad, so I change the subject.

– *What sport do you play?*
– I would like to dance but I do not have a partner.
– *You do not have a partner?*
– I don't have a regular partner. Boys are not that interested in dancing.
– *What dance: classical?*
– Ballroom dancing, also mambo – fun dance.
– *Fun? Is that important in dance?*
– Yes. You move, you are spinning, and you have a pretty shiny dress.
– *Talk about this a little more: you are spinning in a pretty shiny dress.*
– It is a lot of fun. I really enjoy it; everything is okay then.

Martha mentions enjoyment and fun again, in relation to this new topic: dancing.

– *And that you do not have a partner?*
– That really sucks. The boys in my class don't like dancing. And I don't want to dance with older boys. There are two older guys who do not have partners but I don't want to dance with them, as they just go there because they have nothing else to do.
– *They just go there? Why do you go?*
– I go so I can learn the technique.
– *Learn the technique?*
– So I can spin nicely.
– *What would it be like to spin nicely?*
– I would be happy that I could do something with great skill. That would be neat.

The question here is to decide whether the "skilled" or the "happy" is more important: which one is the tool and which one is the goal, the experience of the vital sensation?

– *Did you want to get skilled at the sports you played, too?*
– Yes, of course. But it was not good. I did not improve because

I could not go every day. I did not have the time. The teacher did not care so much about me for this reason, or maybe he just did not like me. He was really strict. When I left he said he was sorry because I had potential.

– *And you?*

– Oh, great. Once in a lifetime they praise me. I am sorry, that's it – I didn't say it to the teacher, just to myself. It does not matter now anyhow. I had another friend there. I really liked her. She was very cheerful.

– *Cheerful?*

– And funny.

– *Are there other people who are cheerful and funny?*

– Many of my classmates. That is why I like school. You can laugh there a lot.

– *Do you also laugh a lot at home?*

– Only if I am watching a funny movie; otherwise, I don't. Or when I am on the phone with my best friend and she tells me funny things.

– *What do you do when you are with her?*

– We do something we call "total silliness." We sit in front of the TV and we turn the volume down and we dub it. So we are saying different things than what they normally do. This sounds extremely funny. The character is serious and we are saying something different.

> Martha, when talking about funny things, uses the same hand motion twice: she lifts her hands and laughs.

– *What is your experience when you do this dubbing with the TV?*

– If we do it right, it does not fit there at all and then it is funny.

– *Does not fit?*

– Something funny comes out of it. Others would laugh, too. It is very cool.

– *I want to understand how is it for you. If I were playing too, I would have to say something that does not fit and then it would be cool?*

– Something that seems to match with the character but does not really. I cannot explain it; you need to feel it. You have to try to guess what he says, but still something very different will be the end result.

— *What is that like?*

— We laugh a lot. It is a game.

— Is this the opposite of "there is nothing?"

— When I am in good relationship with those I love, that's good for me.

> At this point Martha confirms what I have assumed until now: she turns the topic to her relationships and we find out that the "there is nothing" is somehow related to those she loves.

— *And if you're not in good relationship?*

— That is because they do not care about me. I do not like that. I don't have anything to do, anybody to be with if there is nobody there.

> As she is speaking, Martha reveals something very significant through her physical mannerisms. Until now she has been holding one hand with the other, but when she says, "I don't have anything to do, anybody to be with," her two hands suddenly move apart as if she tore something apart. This gesture is similar to the tearing hand gesture she used early in the interview while talking about washing her hair. That's when she made a sudden pulling motion, saying, "there is nothing." And then she went on to relate her hair falling out to her best friend. So the problem becomes clear even on the psychological-symbolic level: the hair loss symbolizes the impossibility, the tearing apart of the relationship. But Martha does not talk about this, a mineral theme, but rather about how "there is nothing" on one hand and, on the other hand, everything is good: fun, enjoyable, cheerful, exciting. This means she experiences this situation in a "plant" way.

— *You do not have anybody to be with. They do not care about you?*

– This does not happen very often. But, for example, if I fight with my best friend, that is not good. That is very bad.

– *What do you fight about?*

– Misunderstandings.

– *Can you give me an example and how you felt about it?*

– I did not say anything and her life just went on, because she has other friends, too. Usually she is fine; everything is good for her.

Her reaction is that she does not talk.

– *Why?*

– She can afford leaving someone. But I do not want to say anything bad about her; I really love her. It is just that she has other friends besides me whom she likes more than me.

– *More than you?*

– Yes, but she really likes me, too.

– *She can afford leaving others?*

– When I am sad, that bothers her, but not as much as it bothers me. But I don't understand anything anymore.

– *You are doing great! When you have nobody to be with, when you fight over a misunderstanding, that is not good and you do not talk – how is that?*

– Then I have nothing to say. I won't say, "Leave me alone."

– *Why not?*

– Why should I? She will notice or someone will point it out to her, but I do not want to hurt her feelings. I do not want to hurt anybody's feelings. Because afterwards she might say, "Fine, if that's what you think, I won't be your friend anymore." I do not want to hurt anybody but nobody wants to hurt anybody.

– *What do you do when something is really bothering you?*

– I feel really bad.

– *But you do not speak?*

– The problem has to be really big in order for me to talk about it.

– *What is that like?*

– Then nothing matters anymore.

– *What happens after the fight? How do you make peace?*

– Maybe we would not make peace at all. It does not bother her that much that she has one less friend. I also have many friends but it is important for me to have a special friend I love more than the others.

– *A best friend?*

– That is a foothold. It is the same for everybody.

– *Foothold?*

– That is good. I am happy then: I am arranging my room, I make something pretty, I go to the movies with my friend, I go to her house, I sleep over. If we fight I cannot do anything about the fact that she has her other friends with whom she has been friends for longer than with me and she likes them more. It is not my fault I met her later. It is also not my fault that another friend of hers does not want her to make friends with me. She is very jealous, so even though we were good friends for a long time, now we do not spend so much time together because she does not let us.

> This new information about her friendships confirms that Martha needs a plant remedy: if she needed a mineral remedy, she would be elaborating on what she was lacking and what her shortcomings were that prevented her from being good friends. Instead, she says it is not her fault; all the reasons are outside of her.

– *How does this other girl not let you spend time with your best friend?*

– She says nasty things about me. She says I should go away, that I am annoying, that I keep coming here.

> Annoying also is a characteristic of the malarial miasm. Martha keeps going there – just as the head lice keep coming back to her.

– *In recess?*

– Yes. I have to find the point when I can go there. I have a third friend but she is a top athlete so she does not have so much time. I almost do not spend any time with my best friend, because the jealous girl does not let us.

– *So who are you with?*
– With my other friends.
– *Is that not as good?*
– Oh yes, it is. I love them, too. It is just that everybody has a best friend with whom they can laugh the best.

> So the most important aspect of a best friend is that you can laugh with them – again, the same "funny" theme.

– *How does the jealous girl do this not letting you spend time with your best friend?*
– She is happy when I am not there. Behind my back she says things like how good it is that Martha is not here.
– *And you?*
– I got used to it. I used to ask her not to do it because it was really nasty but it is always she who turns out to be more nervous. So I left it at that, so she could do whatever she wanted.

> Again, this is the attitude of the person with malaria miasm: they accept that from time to time they are attacked.

– *Now you cannot be with your best friend at all?*
– No, I cannot. By now I think she does not want it anymore.
– *Why don't you say anything to the jealous girl?*
– I don't want to butt in.
– *Why?*
– They could say I was the intruder.
– *Intruder?*
– I was not, but that's what she invented and she spreads it about me.
– *How do you feel about her inventing this and spreading it about you that you were an intruder?*
– Bad, I cannot deal with it.

> Martha's notion of intruding that she accepts as her attribute that was given to her by others is directly linked to the head lice. They are intruders, parasites.

– When she sends me off I feel really crappy.

– *How does it affect your life that you cannot be with your friend?*

– It is really awful that I cannot be with her even though I like her. We cannot fool around this way.

> Martha's last statement here is accompanied by a hand gesture: one hand holding the other. Now she lets it go.

– *You cannot fool around?*

– If we do not do anything for a long time when we are together, she goes off on her own and I am left behind. But this is not her fault. It is not fun to be serious; there is no point to it. I am serious when there is nothing. Sometimes I even laugh when there is nothing, but that's not the real thing.

– *What about the real thing?*

– That's fun and funny.

Finally I ask Martha about her favorite book and movie and what she likes in these areas. She mentions a few favorites, like *Peter Pan* and *Zorro*. She says that she liked these because they were fantasies – exciting and funny – the positive polarity of her sensation.

After my session with Martha is over, I talk again to her mother over the phone. I ask her to tell me more about her daughter: her demeanor, how she reacts to difficulties. She first asks me if I noticed that Martha was making funny faces into the camera I had used to record the session. I told her I had not noticed it during the interview, but later, as I was watching the video, I was stumped to see her twinkling, winking and grimacing into the camera and I wondered how I could have missed it during the interview. Martha's mother tells me that her daughter had done this on purpose, and that she made those funny faces when I did not look at her for a few seconds because I was taking notes. Martha told her mother that it would be amusing for me to watch the video and see those funny faces.

I interpret this as Martha's way of showing her rebelling against the video recording. At the same time, she was conveying something important to me that she could not express with words. These funny faces, and her comment that it would be amusing for me, are now something that I have to take into consideration when picking her remedy. I ask her mother if Martha tended to make funny faces at other times, and her mom tells me that it was in her blood: acting and miming are second nature to her. She was a great hit in the school talent show.

Her mother goes on to explain that Martha is not interested in serious things; she is a mischievous girl, a joker. When I ask her to clarify this, she says, "Clowning, bouncing, acting and being funny. That's how she attracts attention, in a frivolous way. Lightly, with great humor and wit, without philosophy or analyzing."

I give Martha the remedy Piper nigrum: black pepper. In Dr. Sankaran's Sensation Method, the sensations of the Piperaceae (Pepper family) are pain, ennui, boredom and lack of excitement on one hand, and, on the other hand, amusement, cheerfulness and hilarity. The passive reactions to these sensations are boredom, dullness and indolence, and the active reactions are desire for amusement, amelioration by entertainment, dancing, partying and music. The person needs these diversions – the liveliness and mirth. Because the Sensation Method is rather young, there are some gaps that homeopaths are working to fill in. One of these gaps is the lack of a particular remedy for the malarial miasm in the Piperaceae family. Piper nigrum belongs to the sycotic miasm, which is one of the elements of the malarial miasm. That's why I choose this remedy: it is not only very close to the ideal remedy for her, it also includes among its characteristic symptoms "problems in girls in puberty" and, in its mental symptoms, a "lonely, abandoned, friendless state".

Martha takes the remedy in 200c potency. Soon after taking the remedy, her mood changes for the better. Two weeks later the lice are falling out dead from her hair. At this point she becomes ill, runs a fever, has a sore throat and could not get out of bed for a few days. Without consulting me, her mother gives Martha another dose of the remedy. In retrospect, her choice is a good decision. Even in such trivial situations, however, it is important to ask the homeopath's opinion regarding repetition of the dose. Martha recovers by the following day and does not need a repetition in the next six months.

Martha keeps improving, with some small ups and downs, in all areas of her life. "It is like a dream," her mother says. "It is like when a small part that was missing (and in Martha's situation caused her to become out of sorts) got back to its place. Martha is in place. She sleeps very well. She started a new way of conditioning: she is bouncing and doing flips on a trampoline. Most of the time we are having a good time. From time to time she has tough moments but when those pass it is much more pleasant to be with her than before. We can find the common language now."

Two months after the initial dose, Martha's mother calls me to tell me that she feels like a process has begun in a positive direction but that she thinks Martha needs a booster. Eventually we agree that we will wait, without repeating the remedy, unless her chief complaint, the head lice, comes back. Sometimes Martha's mood takes a dip, but in many areas of her life positive changes have occurred: she can mix in better, she can look at herself with critical eyes, she can even bear it if someone else is criticizing her. Now she can laugh at herself, which was unheard of before. She can rise above problems. She's got some perspective and has loosened up. Her skin tone has improved, she takes walks and generally is becoming more active and getting stronger. Everything is peaceful.

Her mother's attitude also has changed towards Martha, which has helped the healing process a great deal. Now she accepts that Martha's interest is not in serious things like books or sports that require great effort, but rather in light, cheerful aspects of life. Her mother also accepts that Martha's approach is emotional: if she does not like an era in history and finds a particular event horrendous, she stops studying and switches off her intellectual curiosity and responsibility. Once, while I was talking with Martha's mother about the positive effects of homeopathic treatment, I had mentioned that this remedy could help us to understand Martha better since knowing the attributes of her homeopathic remedy enables us to see more clearly how the sensations that reside deep inside are Martha's own. This lets us look into her inner world, which in turn can bring about positive changes in our interactions with her. If we recognize that her core sensation is cheerful, jolly and amusing, as opposed to boring and a feeling of "there is nothing," and that her approach to the world is through emotions rather than intellect, then we also acknowledge that rather than embracing a competing style of sport, dance fits her better – or even bouncing and doing flips, which she picked herself after taking the remedy. Dance is not less serious than any other sport, and Martha has a chance to do it seriously but lightly and successfully. If her family understands this, it will be easier for them to support her in finding activities, hobbies and even a career that fit her core characteristics. When her family understands her, it also will be easier to avoid hardships and problems with Martha because they can predict her reactions.

This is an aspect of homeopathy that is not often mentioned: with the help of homeopathic remedies, understanding ourselves and our family members can become more profound. Then it becomes easier to accept others or our own unexpected, peculiar reactions and behaviors. It also becomes easier to find activities that minimize frustration, paving the way to achieve self-expression.

CHAPTER 4

A DEEPER UNDERSTANDING OF THE ANIMAL KINGDOM

Animals are largely characterized by their place in the food chain. One animal is stronger than some other animal, and it can eat that weaker animal or expel it from its territory. But at the same time, that stronger animal is also weaker than some other animal that is one step higher in the food chain. So not only does this initial animal have to deal with strategies to eat the weaker one, it also has to protect itself against the stronger one. Thus, in our Materia Medica, animal remedies are characterized by the sensation of feeling weaker or stronger than other outside forces. People in this category will view reality in terms of me in opposition to you or someone else. Some people will experience this dynamic as a constant sense of being the victim, while others will always feel like the stronger one, the aggressor. Some people will alternate between the two roles in different situations This duality is very characteristic of the animal kingdom. Animals are also territorial creatures. They often belong to a family, a pack, a flock or school. People who need these remedies will often feel obliged to be part of a group and suffer the consequences. But since it is a basic survival urge to belong to the group, it will be important for them.

Some human expressions of territorial feelings are jealousy and envy. Many animal remedies deal with these issues. When talking about their sensations, people will not talk about their inner structure, as minerals do, nor about the effects of the environment on them, as plants do, but their whole person affected by, attacked by, made vulnerable by another entity, be it a headache, depression, their own family members or the weather.

At a deep level of talking about these sensations, these people will describe a dreamland that exists only in their world. They themselves have no idea how they reached that level, but some pictures, images or scenes form in their mind when describing what seems to be the original environment of the animal their remedy is made of.

Before we examine the cases of the animal kingdom, I want to revisit a key component of the Sensation Method of homeopathy so we can see how it applies to the following examples. The power of homeopathic case-taking lies in the fact that it does not involve the emotional layer. As I have mentioned before, our goal as homeopaths is not to explore the emotional layer, nor even the layer that feeds the emotions. Our goal is to arrive at the sensation level and hear the words that describe that level. As we are humans, and homeopathy utilizes our ability to verbalize our feelings, sensations and experiences, we use words to transfer these ideas. But beyond the actual words the coherency of speech has only secondary importance. Describing sensations is often far from what the person is used to. It is far from the realm the ego feels attached to or protective of. Our ego is what works the "pain body," as Eckhart Tolle calls it. With the Sensation Method we go beyond this body and thus trick the ego.

Once the ego has no access to what we are talking about, we can truly describe our core problem with no pain and suffering. There is no guard invested in keeping the pain body as intact as possible. This pain body is the very obstacle to health. Our ego does not want us to be free of it. It wants us to stay ill-healthed because that is its only chance for survival. This process has a dual benefit. First, we can reach the core problem without touching painful, tender spots in the whole being – we don't have to stir up traumatic experiences. Second, upon reaching the core level, we touch something truly essential, and once that essential core is addressed and healed, healing will emanate into the whole being, transforming the whole into a healthy state.

Longing for the Warm Seas of the Caribbean

Elsa, a woman in her 60s, is part of a bilingual women's clinic where she helps less fortunate women to make their own decisions in their health care. That is where I meet her. Elsa impresses me as a powerful, cheerful and very friendly, outspoken woman. As we talk at a professional conference, she tells me that she has always been interested in homeopathy but has not pursued it because in the midst of taking care of others, she keeps neglecting her own needs. She quickly makes an appointment with me for the following week.

As she walks into my office, Elsa looks at a chakra chart on the wall and points at it.

– I like strong colors; those are my colors! I really like red. I just recently knitted this ruby red scarf.

She shows off a decorative scarf she is wearing. She has a strong, dynamic voice and talks fast.

– I always wanted constitutional homeopathic treatment. Once I made an appointment with a homeopath but they could not provide a time that suited me so I said, "Forget about it!" I need a highly reciprocal relationship, so I decided that person was not for me. Then at one of the clinics I worked at, I had a colleague who was also a homeopath. I did not want to go to see her, as we were colleagues. Then, by chance, I met you. So here I am. But it is not a chance, Ildiko, not a chance. There are many things that are somehow determined – people come into your life on purpose. And you have to make the decision on the spot. You say, "I will do it."

Hints for the animal kingdom are emerging as soon as Elsa starts talking. She speaks in an energetic and animated way. When telling her story she does not start from her aches and pains but rather her previous encounters with homeopaths. The way she recalls those experiences is not related to her inner strength, abilities or structural issues, as in a mineral case. It is not about a plant's sensitivity either. It is about her encounters with people who did not suit the kind of relationship she expected. It was the way they related to her that affected her.

– *How can I help you.*

– I am healthy; I have no major health issues. I am a person who is very much connected to earth. I do not take medications. If I get a headache that turns awful and I need to work, I take a Tylenol®. I cannot say I am in bad health but I do have little aches and pains here and there. I know I could be much more balanced, to be in better health. I suffer from the climate here in the North. Soon I am planning to go back to the Caribbean. It is nice and warm there, so I will be less cold there, I know. I lived in South America for twenty-five years. I need to go back there. It is horribly cold here! I hate it! But I have to be here for now. Here in this cold weather I always have cold feet, and I hate to have cold feet! I hate it, hate it! When my neighbors come over they always say how hot it is in my house. So I am wondering if my body is functioning correctly.

> I am avoiding using exclamation marks after each of her statements here, though it feels like each one is an exclamation. Her cheery disposition and positive attitude quickly fills the room, sweeping me off into her world. There is a flow of associations between each segment of her story, though sometimes it might be not obvious at first glance.

– The other physical problem I have is recurrent vaginal infections, even when I am not sexually active. It comes on and off. What else can I tell you… I am a true Gemini. I am in two worlds. It is too fast-paced here for me. This is a workaholic country. I decided to move here because my daughter lives here. I was born in Denmark during the war. When I was eight I took care of my two younger sisters. My mom is old and sickly now so I have taken up the role of mom for her.

I am very creative. I am never bored. I do projects, explorations. I am interested in anthropology.

> I notice that she is curling up in the chair, hugging her arms tight around her chest and sides. I point this out to her.

– Oh, yes. I like to be in the fetal position. I love that position. Even before I did Reiki I used to use the energy of my hands. When I was a nurse I used to touch the patients. Touch is very important, you know. I find that when I get a little pain somewhere, I place my hands there and the warmth and the energy heals the sore spot.

– *Say more about the fetal position.*

– Warmth comes from my hands. It goes through my skin to the inner organs. If I painted it I would paint short lines like this

> She shows horizontal lines one above the other.

– I am connected to water! I like nice warm water. That is why I love the Caribbean. I also take nice warm baths a lot. I love to snorkel, too. Now my hands warmed me up too much. My whole body got warm.

> Notice how she comes to the warm sea through energetic description. She arrives at it through her position that is a non-verbal expression of her inner experience, especially because she often resorts to this position. She describes her sensation with lines of an abstract shape in a potential painting. It is a valuable inner image, a straightforward expression of her energy, bypassing explanations of the emotional and mental realms.

– *Tell me more about the feeling in the warm bath.*

– Oh, it is like heaven! When I go home I start the bath. Just hearing the water makes me hayayayay... I want to go in there. When I am in the bath I often fall asleep; I feel so good. I love water! Since I was a child I have loved water. I have a baby picture where I am splashing in a little pool! I learned to swim very early. Every summer I was swimming. The North Sea was very cold, but I did not know anything else. Then, when I first went to Puerto Rico, I knew I loved the Caribbean! I love the people there, the way people are. I love the water there, with those colors: the blue, the turquoise. Sometimes it is contaminated. I do not like that.

Once I had the most beautiful experience with a dolphin. The fishermen told me there was a dolphin that came to shore sometimes, but not often. It was my last day there and we were on a beach with my daughter. I was swimming. My daughter suddenly started waving to me, all scared because a dolphin was approaching. I think she thought it was a shark. So I just waved back to her that it was okay. The dolphin came towards me and we played. As I swim very well I started following the dolphin. He – or she, I am not sure what it was – just went off deeper in the sea. I went after him, went after him, went after him. I would not have turned back if not for my daughter's call. I realized when my daughter called how far out I had gone!

Why did I do that? I do not know. As I was swimming there, my head under the water, it was beautiful! Maybe the most beautiful experience I ever had with nature! Why did I follow the invitation? I have no idea. I just did it. I felt comfortable, had a lot of trust. I am not terribly fearful. In Puerto Rico the crime rate is high. I have a good nose for danger form living there so long. I am street-wise. I learned to live with scary situations. Apart from that I am not fearful. Torture could change quite a bit but in normal circumstances I am not afraid.

– *Are there any animals you are afraid of?*

– Yes. Snakes. And I don't like mosquitoes. I was not afraid of dogs, but then I had a bad experience with one in Puerto Rico. One day walking home from the beach a German shepherd bit me in the back. It wasn't so much the dog but the owner. She did not even say she was sorry. She should have taken me to the hospital. Now I do not like German shepherds. I always talk to animals.

– *You talk to animals?*

– Yes. Well, I don't talk to mosquitoes. I talk to houseplants, too. They grow better when I talk with them.

– *Describe again the sensation when you were swimming out in the ocean after the dolphin.*

– The water was very nice and warm. I had to swim after the dolphin. I had to! It was a silent invitation. I felt so not afraid. Maybe there were sharks but I was not afraid of anything. I was trusting. I knew nothing would happen to me. If anything, that animal would protect me. The fishermen told me that once somebody hit that dolphin on the nose. I thought, God, how can anybody do such a cruel thing?! No wonder he (or she) was not coming to the shore anymore.

> In Elsa's encounters with animals we see interesting use of language. She blames the owner of the dog rather than the dog for biting her. People who need animal remedies often talk as if looking at humans from an outsider's perspective. She also expresses a similar feeling when talking about the dolphin and the people who cruelly hit his nose. Again, she is looking at humans from the outside, and their actions seem to be foreign to her. It is commonly seen in animal cases when the person talks about "humans."

– *Describe that you are being in two worlds.*

– First of all, I mean it in a cultural sense. Perhaps I was meant to move from Denmark to Puerto Rico. They are culturally two different worlds. I love Afro-Caribbean dance. Once a dance teacher told me that in Europe you dance like in a cathedral and in the Caribbean it is wavy like the sea!

> Elsa follows this statement with large, wavy gestures of her arms.

– I travel between these two worlds. I embraced the spiritual side, which comes from the Afro-Caribbean religions. I learned about trusting destiny. In Denmark it would be called superstition!

> She laughs.

Getting to know indigenous cultures made me less westernized. That's how indigenous cultures affect you! I wanted to learn how they saw the world.

> She is describing her reality that is divided into two different worlds. She is very outspoken about the spiritual, the "Caribbean" side, but I also have to understand the "Scandinavian" side. Animal remedies often have a split; they talk about two sides within themselves. Elsa mentions being a true Gemini and the two cultures she carries within herself.

– *Tell me more about you as a child.*

– I was born during the war. My father disappeared and my mother left us to go to search for him. She was gone for nine months. Meanwhile, I was well taken care of. She left me with my aunts and other extended family. There were a lot of people around me in my first and second year. My aunt caused a phobia in me, though! I cannot stand hot cereal. Just thinking about it can make me gag and throw up. Smelling it is even worse! She used to pinch my nose closed so I would open my mouth. I have a nose phobia, too. I cannot bear for my nose to be touched by anyone. My father's side of the family is very intellectual. Mother's side is more affectionate.

I was a redhead, so the other kids made fun of me. They called me "heks" – that's Danish for witch. I laugh at it now, because that's what I am! I am a good witch. I had a nice, free childhood. I roamed around the streets. I was not afraid of anything. I loved taking care of my little sister. I was a little slow in my studies. My teacher used to hit kids, and he hit me once. And I was not at fault. I felt it was truly unjust!

I am very keen on injustice. My father was a judge, so maybe it runs in the family. Social justice for me is a fundamental thing in life. I met that teacher twenty-some years later. I saw him on the street from behind and recognized his gait. When he turned around I saw his face. He was much older, of course, but I recognized that gait. I saw his back at the blackboard so much.

I told him about my life, about my teaching. I told him there was one thing I do not do to my students: I never hit them. And I told him I remembered that he did. He felt so terribly bad, he almost fainted. It seems like he had blocked it out completely. I told him I did not even deserve the punishment. That experience taught me I would never be unjust to another person! I was a very active, courageous child. It changed when I was fourteen and we moved to southern Denmark, to a small provincial town. My father was the only judge there and we were strangers. We spoke a different dialect and were also Protestants, as opposed to the majority of that town. We were shunned but also somewhat respected there. I went to fashion school, then to nursing. I decided on that because there was a bad nurse shortage. I was much more into psychology, not surgical nursing. I believed that you needed to talk to the patient. As a young nurse my primary job was to clean all the time, not to talk to the patients. I was part of the Protestant Nurses' Association and we decided that we could not go on like this. As a spokesperson for the group I went to the director. You have to understand that he was at a very-very high position, the ultimate authority. A nurse student would never ever talk to him! And I got so sick from this; I got gastritis! Later I dealt much better with authorities.

> The trigger for animal remedies is when they feel weaker than their opponent – there is someone above them who is stronger, more powerful, and they have to deal with that. Being weaker or stronger, winning or losing, being the victim or the aggressor – these are the main triggers for animal remedies. Elsa gets a serious physical ailment from this encounter. She feels very strongly about certain issues in the hospital, so strong that she feels compelled to speak up, even if she has to face the highest authority. The prospect of developing an adverse physical reaction does not stop her either. In this example we can see the strength of such an urge, truly a force of survival. The quality of

the remedy source, the animal's instinctive behavior, translates into human actions.

– I got married and moved to Puerto Rico with my husband. Four years later I divorced him. Once I decide on something, nobody can convince me otherwise!! I get to an inner last point and there is no way back. And I am articulate about it. I am very honest. Some people do not like it. I think it is important to share with another person what you feel. It is about sharing perceptions. Trust is a must for me! With my husband, the problem was that the longer we lived together the more machismo came out of him! I was dependent on him. I didn't speak Spanish. He worked; I did not. But eventually I said I did not come here to be a little housewife! And he was not supportive of my independence. Things really got rotten. At some point I became submissive. I felt I gave up my true being. I was defeated. I had been outgoing before. At one point I lost it, became intimidated. I lost trust in myself. But then I turned back again into that courageous girl I used to be!

The low point in her life comes as she is defeated into submission.

– I have a very good relationship with my daughter. She is thirty-one now. We share trust, a lot of trust. I don't trust her father anymore. I was alone; he didn't want me to go out. You have to grow a lot, overcome obstacles, be creative and assimilate to the culture you live in. He did not understand all that. We lived like in a ghetto. I always thought you had to learn the language, and then you could have opinions. First you had to learn the culture. You cannot judge it right away. So after the divorce I really plunged into the local life. I have my family now in the many, many friends I made. They are my family.

– *Tell me about your relationships with your friends.*

– They are my base. They create an affectionate environment and make it humanistic. There are certain principles involved. Solidarity is very important. A real friend is the one that is there for you when you really need them. Friendship is a two-way street.

I am affectionate. I like to kiss, hug, hold hands with my patients or with people. I look you in the eye. I feel when there is good vibration. I like touch. I am a touching, embracing midwife.

> I feel she is taking the course of her story to a direction
> that does not bring us closer to her vital sensation, so
> I ask her a question that gives her the opportunity to
> talk about something that is not intellectualized and
> gives me a broad view on reality as she sees it.

— *Say more about your life in Puerto Rico.*

— I worked there as a midwife assisting in home births. Often I had to go to houses at night, so I often found myself walking on the streets at 3 a. m. I was very watchful. I couldn't care less about material things, but I would never ever let anybody rape me! Sometimes I would sense that a car was following me, but for some reason the guy decided that I was not the one. I sensed it.

> She keeps coming back to situations of danger, of
> hierarchy, of the interplay between weaker and
> stronger.

— *Tell me about sensing things.*

— I am clairvoyant. Once a very good friend of mine was dying of AIDS. I was walking on the street and suddenly I felt a very strong, sudden sensation: bummm. It hit me right in the heart. When I went home there was a message on my phone from his brother. I called him back and he told me my friend just passed half an hour ago — the same time I felt that strong sensation. Three days later I was supposed to go to a midwifery conference. I was considering canceling it, because of his death. I was hesitating for a long time but then I decided I had to go. I heard his voice saying, "Go! Of course you have to go. It is very important that you go to this retreat." And true, it turned out to be a life-changing event for me. I did not have these clairvoyant moments in Denmark. It came out in Puerto Rico. That was the environment where this could come out.

— *Tell me about your decision-making process.*

— Before the decision there is uncertainty. You go back and forth in your head. Then you say to yourself, "It is now or never." Once you make that decision it is the feeling of well-being and freedom. The pressure is all gone; the whole body relaxes.

> She opens her arms wide and smiles with apparent relief.

– I know I need to listen to my body. It also happened last April, when I had to make a big decision. My body was breaking out: I had many pains, aches, rashes, boils and herpes. I knew my body was trying to tell me something and I had to listen! Once I made the decision I felt calm and free. I was sure I was doing the right thing. I was not sure how it was going to work out but I knew it was gonna be all right! I trusted my body.

> She talks about this experience the same way she talks about the experience with the dolphin. It is a complex sensation, which points to the animal kingdom. The characteristic of it is that she sees two entities: herself and the other self (or the dolphin in the previous example). Even though the situation is unclear or even dangerous she decides to trust her instinct and follow that other voice. This decision brings her great relief and a sensation of freedom. Having two sides and a split between the two is often seen in animal remedies.

– *How does it feel when you are calm and sure it is gonna be all right?*
– The body feels like in tune with what your mind says. It is a beautiful bonding of mind and body. Everything is coming together.

> She shows this with a gesture of interlocking fingers. This sensation causes the two to merge. The sensation of the compensated state is a relief for people who need animal remedies. Often these are moments when they experience the healing of the split.

– It is like when I look out of the window and see the sky, the blue sky and the waves turning like this.

> She makes wavy hand gestures.

It is harmony. It is the way you want it to be. The way it is supposed to be. Even though I know life is not always blue I feel ready to whatever comes along. A metaphor for it that I love is open doors. I never lock my doors. I do not like shut doors or closed windows. In Puerto Rico people have iron rods on their windows. I don't! I am not gonna live in a prison! Besides, I have a baseball bat next to my bed and I have very good ears. I sense it right away if anybody is coming! If someone puts a ladder there and tries to climb up into my room with bad intentions, I would have no qualms about pushing that ladder away or using that baseball bat. That is my self-defense! I am very protective of myself and my privacy. Don't you dare touch me when I have not invited you! I mean a hostile touch. Don't you dare because I can react very forcefully! People do not think I am capable of doing it, but I am very determined! I have no second thoughts about that. I have a very good sensation about what is hostile and what is not. I would not make a mistake about that!

> At this level the animal qualities of Elsa's case are clearly shining through. The main sensation is that of survival of the fittest: being the victim or the aggressor is what counts. There is not only one sensation running through the whole case that would determine a plant remedy. She does not see herself as one in need of improving her structure, performance or relationships. After determining that she needs an animal remedy, the subkingdom and the specific animal need to be found. Elsa talks frequently about being part of a group. She stands up for the group of young nurses in Denmark, she calls her colleagues her midwife sisters and she feels her extended family is what is so valuable for her in Puerto Rico. Being part of a group is a characteristic of the mammals. Also, she has nurturing tendencies and has found her true vocation in midwifery. She mentions the "most beautiful encounter" she has had with nature in the form of

swimming with the dolphin. Not only is she demonstrating qualities of the animal kingdom and specific characteristics of mammals, but she has talks about the very issues that have come up that point to the remedy made out of dolphin's milk. So, at this visit, Elsa receives a dose of Lac delphinum 200c, the remedy made of the milk of the dolphin.

ABOUT THE REMEDY LAC DELPHINUM

Homeopathic remedies are born by going through a process called proving. First, the remedy is made: in this process the original crude substance is diluted and potentized according to the rules of homeopathic remedy-making. For the remedy Lac delphinum, a drop of dolphin milk was used as the original substance. The dilution process minimizes the actual crude substance to a degree where there is not one molecule of the original substance found in the remedy. Nevertheless, the remedy carries the energetic blueprint of the substance. Once the remedy is ready, it is given to a group of volunteers from whom data is collected: their mental, emotional and physical reactions to the remedy. Once this data is collected it is organized, and symptoms that arise in several individuals are arranged by themes. Proving is our first look into the inner life of an otherwise latent substance. Later, as the remedy is used in clinics all around the world, the information grows and gets enhanced by the characteristics of people who were helped by it.

The dolphin milk has a relatively recent proving. It was conducted by Nancy Herrick[7] in Maui, Hawaii. The main themes of the remedy came up very strongly in several provers (people

---

[7] Herrick, Nancy, *Animal Mind, Human Voices, Provings of Eight New Animal Remedies.* Nevada City, CA: Hahnemann Clinic Publishing (1998)

who take the remedy during the proving process). The most prominent characteristic is the feeling of calmness despite danger. This can be linked to the fact that dolphins live in protective pods. They love to play and enjoy physical contact with one another. Their main predator, the shark, lurks around the pod in hungry search for calves. The calves are kept in the middle of the pod for protection but the survival rate to adolescence is still rather low. The danger is a strong element in a dolphin's life but it does not lessen their playful essence.

This description fits Elsa in that she has a cheerful, playful personality but, on the other hand, she seeks groups where she can belong. She is no stranger to danger, either. One of the first things she mentions about Puerto Rico is that she learned how to be street wise, so despite danger she would worked, and walk around at night. She also mentions how she felt safe in the middle of possible danger when following the dolphin in the sea. The fact that she refuses to put iron bars on her window but keeps a baseball bat handy reinforces this theme.

The feeling of being separated comes from the proving. Elsa's feeling of being separate from the group surfaced when she moved to the little provincial town as a child and later when she suffered living "in a ghetto" in Puerto Rico. She seems to crave the company of larger groups, communities – the way dolphins gather in pods.

According to the proving, people who need Lac delphinum are clairvoyant. Elsa refers to several occasions where her clairvoyance played an important role in her decision-making.

The interesting thing about the source of this remedy is that it is made of the Bottlenose dolphin. Elsa makes several references to her sensitive nose; she uses the word nose in metaphors as well. As she says, she has a "nose phobia." And the dolphin she meets at sea was injured in his nose. The Bottlenose dolphin received its name because of the distinctive shape of its snout that looks like a bottle.

Follow-up visit, 6 weeks later:

– I am curious to know what remedy you gave me! I feel good, tremendous. A major change is coming to my life: I decided to retire. I am retiring from this country, not just from my job! I feel a process is finished, a new phase starting. The remedy seems to have come at a right moment. Maybe the reason I came to see you was that I sensed that change was about to happen. Maybe the remedy has helped me to realize this change. I feel tremendous. I am going home to Puerto Rico. I was there two weeks ago and visited my daughter. She is in an identity crisis so I said I had to go there to see her. We discussed many serious things about her life. I talked to my ex-husband, too. There is some trauma between them, but it is not my job to sort it out. It was important to talk to them. It was a wonderful homecoming. In Spanish you say pisatiera: touch down. I feel I touched down because I am going home.

Physically I feel very, very energized. I can see a little bit from above. I see that in my clinic. Yesterday I talked to them and gave them some suggestions for the future. I think that was my contribution to this place. I am a very dedicated person. I love my work, and I worked hard and with passion here. Now, as I am retiring I can see things from a different perspective, which I think should be valuable for those who stay here. I see very clearly what I want to do. I am a very happy person right now. I have clear thoughts about many things: I feel good, very clear in my head.

– *What about your physical symptoms? Any change there?*

– I told you about the cold in my extremities. It has been better. About the animals: I have been visited by a red robin and two dogs. I looked the dog in the eyes and spoke Spanish to him. I like to be with people.

I had some serious discussions with my daughter and some friends and colleagues. It felt so good. That's what I felt; I had to do it. That's closed now. I needed to do it, and when I am on that path nobody can tell me to change! That is the feeling: that I have had clarity.

– *Any other physical symptoms?*

– I have had some numbness in my lips, where I had herpes in the past. After taking the remedy there was a small outbreak and it is gone now. The crust on my nose is getting smaller. It is better, too. The vaginal infection came mildly once. I have to keep watching that, because it tends to come and go. I am not tired during the day; I feel more energized and I do not need as much sleep as before. I got some red wine and did not have any migraine from it!

The big decision I talked to you about last time was about giving up my job. I feel it is too much. I feel if I do not give up this job I am going to break apart. The situation is so rotten. We are not respected. You are an abused victim, and I cannot take that! I am not going to be like that – to be trampled upon! And I feel that there is a new direction looking in my face. I have new project ideas in mind, creative things! I know that when you are passionate about a project you make others passionate, too. I have that ability.

When I went to see my dentist he said I took such good care of my teeth. Usually I have to go to see him every three months because I have an infection in my gums. He said my teeth looked splendid! There was no infection. It is unusual.

– *Any dreams recently?*

– I had a dream about dolphins.

> The right action to take in situations when the person is improving is to wait. There is no need to repeat the remedy. The dose did its job and Elsa is healing on her own. Follow-up interviews are needed to determine when the next dose is necessary. When someone is improving mentally and emotionally, as well as physically, these follow-up visits can be stretched further apart.
>
> Six months later Elsa returns for her next visit. She has had an eventful six months and tells me all about it! She talks about all her trips to exotic places, encounters with interesting people, colorful assemblies, thought-

provoking seminars and inspiring conferences. She describes all the chance encounters with people in different cities who had acquaintances at other places she visited or were part of events she was planning to go to. She made connections, good friends, and in general felt she was going in the right direction. She recounts how in the previous year she had tried to plan her trips and now in these past few months she went with the flow.

– I am so very happy! And I feel very relaxed about it all.

She talks about an assembly in New York called Doctors for Global Health. She decided on the spur of the moment to go and while there she saw a video on Guatemala, a beautiful documentary. She made connections with like-minded doctors and soon found herself traveling for causes she believed in.

– I feel great. It had to happen this way. I feel part of the community. I had someone close to me getting into a bad situation: she was kidnapped, drugged and raped. This touched me deeply. But I know my antennas are high. I feel the vibrations. I am prepared for situations like that. I would fight. There are specific ways to talk and behave. I also learned self-defense. You need to fight. Do not show fear. Otherwise, they finish you. If there are many people it is more difficult but with one person you can do it.

People all over Latin America have disappeared. This is politics. Horrible things have happened there. People who believed in freedom or who belonged to an organization disappeared. For many years I also had a file. Just because I want to live free. This makes me stronger, gives me calmness. I feel what I do is right. People ask me how can I still be so optimistic. Well, if you are ingrained and despairing you cannot do anything; you are paralyzed! Many people live in a denying way, that they do not care what happens to the rest of the world. They want to be safe and secure. I will never be that way. Being a judge was a mission for my father.

He lived "Justice for all," And I think I got it from him. He said when he was dying, "I will live within you children, when I die." I felt after he passed that a part of his soul came into me. It was a beautiful September morning. His soul was accompanied by the birds' chirping and the nature around. I really think that a little part of his soul came into me because he was also a poet and a year later I started writing in poetic form. I never did that before. Now, that is interesting... I use the word "accompany" a lot. I recently realized that six years ago I wrote in my introduction on the clinic's website that I am honored to accompany women in their journey to become mothers. At the Assembly I took part in recently we talked a lot about accompanying and community. I realized these are very important for me. Now, as I am talking I am realizing that in all these aspects of my life how crucial this accompaniment and community is for me.

I like the metaphor weaving and knitting. It makes me think of the fishermen nets. We put things together: different colors, a network between people, communities, countries. How we can create a better world by creating a network. My nose is telling me that this is the right way.

> She points to her nose.

I also have a good sense of smell. I love smells, but it is also a metaphor for finding the right people, the right things to go after. I feel everything. It is a component of a healer. With indigenous people, there is such a strong connection.

> Elsa fills up the consultation time without me
> interrupting with any questions. But before she leaves,
> I want to know about her two chief physical symptoms.
> So I ask about the cold feet and the vaginal infections.

– The cold feet were much better until I had the altitude sickness at the Ecuador conference, when I felt so sick. I think it was an emotional drain. My feet were colder again! I cuddled, put socks on. The vaginal infection still comes and goes but it is milder, not so irritating, and does not last as long as before.

Her energy is all expressed in her stories, which indicates the 1M potency. I give her a few doses, instructing her to take it when the vaginal infection returns.

A year later I happened to visit the clinic Elsa had worked at. I was informed that she had retired and moved back to Puerto Rico. I sent her an email asking how she was doing, and she wrote back:

Saludos de Puerto Rico… greetings from Puerto Rico, where I arrived after a three-month visit to Denmark after retiring from the clinic in New York. I am happy to be back in Puerto Rico, even though I miss my midwife sisters, the women and the very special place the clinic is. Thanks to you as my homeopath, my decisions for this important step became even more clear and I really thank you for your great care. I took the remedy once more after the death of my mother last year, when I traveled back and forth from Denmark a couple of times. My health and spirits have been great and I am looking forward to the projects I will be working on. Warm regards, Elsa.

I am happy to close this case with the knowledge that Elsa has found her way back home and is now enjoying the warm seas.

A Case Where Acute and Chronic Matches the Same Remedy

The following case is an example of how an acute situation can bring someone to the homeopath's office and receive a remedy that fits their constitution, the overall characteristics of the person. In the kidney stone case in Chapter 3, we saw a cure for an acute illness. In the absence of long-term follow-up we do not know whether or not the remedy that helped the acute phase was the constitutional remedy or whether it was a true acute situation. Acute illnesses can be categorized into two groups. One is the so-called "true" acutes, where the acute symptoms have nothing in common with the person's chronic weaknesses; they come and go. These symptoms usually arise because the stress they induced in the person is too large for the vital force to shake off without producing symptoms. It can be anything from a physical trauma to the local flu virus. They develop a similar symptom picture in any individual who is affected by them. The other type of acutes is the flare-up of the underlying weakness, therefore exposing the person's constitutional traits. In a true acute situation the person needs a remedy that is different from their constitutional remedy, but in the case of a flare-up the constitutional remedy will help. It will take care of the acute problem and also will bring long-lasting relief of other, seemingly unrelated chronic problems.

> This is what happened in the case of Julia, who suffered from edema and carpal tunnel syndrome during her pregnancy. The recount of her case starts with this email from Julia:

– I am 29 years old, 35 weeks pregnant. I have another good month to go. Last month, around Christmas I noticed that my hands went numb at night with a hot sensation. I told my obstetrician, finding out that it was very common during pregnancy, caused by water retention, and should go away after the baby was born. At that time there was no pain, just mostly discomfort that I could deal with. A few days after I had noticed the numbness I started to feel very sharp pain in my fingers and hands (I think in the bones). I would wake up for the pain about three hours after going to sleep. I did shake my hands, walked around until the pressure and pain felt less, but could only go back to sleep for very short periods, no matter what position I chose. The doctors told me to take Benadryl® or Tylenol®, which I was very upset about, as I was so careful during my whole pregnancy to avoid any medication. I did take Tylenol® once, having no effect on the pain.

Then I was told to see a physical therapist that treated me for carpal tunnel syndrome without success. On her advice I bought a pair of splints, which I thought solved the problem, as the pain was off for a few days. Lately it does not matter if I wear the splints or not; my hands get very puffy, and the pain just does not go away. (The numbness and pressure is now there almost during the whole day.) I spend my nights walking and crying (I think I normally handle pain pretty well.) it takes out all the energy I have, I get depressed, upset, and I don't know where to look for help. I have read about Nux vomica in homeopathy books and on the Internet as well, where it said that pregnant women usually took it for morning sickness, but it also helped with pain associated with water retention. I have purchased and took one dose last night and it seemed to help, but I feel guilty that I have not mentioned it to the obstetrician before taking it. (I just did not feel any effort from their side in listening or really caring.) I feel bad about taking remedies without asking a professional, but I could not go for another night. I feel a lot safer taking the homeopathic products before taking any drugs, knowing a tiny bit about homeopathy, but I do not want to mistreat myself and especially the baby! I am hoping to hear from you soon. Regards, Julia L.

> After I answer Julia's email, she schedules a visit. She
> has a nice, calm demeanor; she does not express as

vivid a personality as Elsa's. Nevertheless, she describes her physical complaints in depth, as her pain is rather acute and she feels desperate to find a natural way to ease it. She flows to the general discussion about her history with ease, without much prompting. As it usually happens with animal remedies she gives a full picture of her personality by referring to stories. There are characters in these stories, often situations of danger and a fight for something.

– *Please describe your symptoms.*

– My right hand is swollen. There is burning pain and numbness in it. It is a hot feeling inside. The pain is worse for pressure; it feels as if it was full of liquid, that there is pressure from the inside. I wake up for the pain at night. I get up, have to move around. I cry all night; it is torturing me. I don't want to take Tylenol®, so as not to hurt the baby. The pain does not stop. I am walking shaking my arms.

– *How are you doing emotionally?*

– I am on a road. This is a road I chose; I am trying to navigate it based on past relationships and mistakes I have made. I have no idea where this road leads me. This relationship and the baby were my decisions, both quick decisions. I must say I did not think it through well. We got married very soon after we met. He asked me to marry him and I decided on the spur of the moment to say yes. Now I am pregnant.

– *What other physical symptoms do you have?*

– When I was a child I suffered from asthma and bronchitis. I remember getting shots for the suffocation. I used to choke when I caught a cold. I had bad colds. More recently I have also noticed that colds and the related choking are connected to my state of mind. It is usually relationships that stress me out. In my last relationship we ended up in court; it was pretty dramatic. I had a lot of choking problems then. Once, in another relationship, the guy's aunt was trying to take us apart with pretty harsh methods. That was also stressful. Colds and flu come when

I am emotionally challenged. Once after a breakup I kept getting colds with suffocation for almost a year. I was on antibiotics for that entire time.

— *Anything else?*

— When I was in high school I had bulimia. I was not happy in any way; I felt out of place. In my childhood I lived with an unfortunate self-image: everybody said I resembled my grandmother a great deal and she was the most hated person in the family! She was a very selfish person. I always wanted to prove that I was not like her, and I knew I was not like her!

I was born in a village in Slovakia. When I was fourteen we moved to a bigger city in Hungary. My country, my environment, the language and all circumstances changed suddenly. The kids were teasing me because of my foreign name, so I came up with a new name and started using that. Everybody told me how to behave, how to live my life. Not even one decision was mine. I didn't feel like making my own decisions anymore. I had to be told where to go, what to do. I was not aware of this. Then I was in a relationship with a guy who told me I had to find myself. He could not continue the relationship because I did not seem to know who I was. He said we were too different. Later I started pulling myself together. I realized that not all my attributes were positive but they were nevertheless mine.

> Julia is telling me her story without stopping. I sit and wait for the opportunity when she says something that carries energy that can lead me deeper into the layers where I will be able to find her remedy. Notice how she uses imagery of fighting: the pain in her hand is torturing her, she fights with feelings, she is in battle with her ego — these are attributes of the animal kingdom. She also recounts a story, similar to Elsa, where she was rendered submissive and lost her real identity. This is a scenario in which animal remedies tend to get stuck.

— *What attributes?*

– Being selfish, for example. First I fought with the feeling that I was similar to my grandmother. What I realized was that everybody was selfish to a certain degree.

– *Please describe this more.*

– I want everything. I prefer receiving than giving. It manifests in everything: standing in line at the grocery store or parking my car. I never liked letting my spot go over to another. I have come a long way in this respect. Now I do not always feel the way I used to, that I am in a fight for territory with another person. It creeps in there, and that is a battle between my ego and me. I am still definitely conscious of this conflict. If I don't fight, if I don't let my ego fight, I can understand the other in a relationship. There are painful experiences but if you try to listen to them you both get less hurt.

> Here, Julia is describing her inner experience: it is about fighting, whether it be two sides of herself, her ego and her; an inner conflict or conflict with the outside; her family or boyfriends; or just people standing in line for groceries. In all of these cases where she feels she is rightfully selfish, she sees the world as being the winner and loser.

– *Describe the ego.*

– The ego wants everything to itself. It wants the beautiful things, the goodies, and wants them fast.

– *Fast? Is "fast" important?*

– Yes. That's how it can get more. If it gets immediately what it wants, it has the capacity to get even more. Through all my romantic relationships I realized that what matters is not how I feel towards my partner, but rather how they react to me. I want to be admired and loved. I have to feel they think I am the one and only for them. That is more important than my feeling this way towards them. My husband had not been planning to get married but when he met me he felt I was the one for him. That played an important role in why I said yes to him. He is scared of becoming a father. His father used to abuse him, humiliated him when he was a kid. He is afraid of what kind of father he is going to be. Things like this come up in our fights.

> I ask her to describe their fights. It is important to know the exact character of her fights because that will help me see what upsets her, how she reacts, in what manner and what is important for her. This is what gives me a glimpse into her inner essence.

– I don't like when he tells me how to do things, when he thinks he knows better than I do. I used to be abrupt and suddenly felt out of control when someone attacked me. Now that I am pregnant I feel the same way but I just burst into tears. I am working hard on keeping up this relationship. I don't want to get to a point when I feel I want to leave him. All the guys I left eventually were begging me to get back together, but I cannot do it. It is a one-time event for me that I fall in love with someone. Once they break that trust there is no return.

> Julia is sensitive to being told what to do, when someone tries to boss her around. Her anger is abrupt, as are her decisions. There is an all-or-nothing feeling in her world. She loves giving it all but once the trust is broken it is gone, quickly and permanently gone. The other aspect she talks about is the need to be admired. She wants her partner to be deeply in love with her, to feel that he considers her to the one and only. These are attributes of the subkingdom within the animal kingdom that is forming here as she goes along in telling her story.

– In my last relationship, he cheated on his wife with me. He was my boss and he started flirting with me. I did not want to get into this type of relationship but I was really attracted to him. We could not stop it. He did not want to divorce his wife, so I knew it would end nasty. He was so conceited; he thought he was in control, that everything was in his hands. He couldn't believe I would ever leave him. Once his wife found out about us we both were fired. I was the first one to find a job. In fact, I was working two jobs while he was unemployed. When he finally got employed I left him; I did not want to leave him while he was without a job. After awhile I went back to him. It was purely sexual attraction, which I have not found in others. But eventually I realized that I was worth more. I needed more. He didn't notice me, didn't pay attention to me. Don't take me wrong; I am not the victim here. That's not how I feel. In a relationship I always try to change the other. I want to change the man into my dream man. I want to shape him; I don't want to change myself.

> She is playing with the opposites here in her description. Therefore, it is meaningful. She describes her relationship with zeal. The image she uses to describe her lover is also a description of the remedy she needs because it is a reflection of reality the way she sees it. She feels like the superior one in the victim–aggressor relationship. She is attracted to this man who fell from his position because of her. Nevertheless, she leaves him because she feels she is worth more. The interplay of these forces is an attribute of the animal kingdom.
>
> I ask her about the word victim as she uses it with emphasis. Her description of this word is meaningful. As I mentioned earlier, the animal kingdom is about seeing reality as a play of two opposing forces. People who need a remedy of the animal kingdom view each element of reality as one that is stronger and one that is weaker; one that wins and one that loses. The tension of opposites builds up the energies of a person. In the expressions of each individual, both extremes can be found and seen. In this case all Julia's relationships are presented as a balancing act between the strong and the weak. The center of the relationship is always sexuality or attraction. In her mind, leaving someone has to be her decision. When she was dumped, when it was not her that decided to separate, she got sick for a whole year. This reaction illustrates

the crucial nature of this dynamic for her. When she tells me that she is not the victim, it means that the victim–aggressor relationship is important for her. Otherwise, she would not mention this word. In some relationships she feels the stronger one and in some the weaker one. Her description of either will give insight into the specific way she views it. This will be our way to see which subkingdom her remedy is from.

– I throw myself into a relationship. I have an ideal picture in my mind and nothing can compare to that. So in each relationship I get less than that ideal. I want caring, true interest in the other. That's how it feels when you fall in love, isn't it?

– *When in love? How does it feel?*

– There is no reality. Every decision seems easy. Nothing is impossible; you can do anything. I made a decision regarding my husband: I am staying with him and any obstacle that comes, we will fight our way through it. This way, reality turns into a fairy tale. In my previous relationship I was so attracted to the guy that it was very hard to decide to leave. It was a very strong attraction. Had he not betrayed me, had he not cheated on me, I would have stayed with him.

In my relationship before him the guy just left me. I was devastated. I had the cold and asthma for a year after that loss. He had asked me to marry him, then he left for home to Brazil and did not seek me. He gave me a month to say goodbye to my family and then I would come after him and we would get married. I kept calling him, and he would not answer. One day he picked up the phone and just said, "Why are you still calling me?" That was a big blow for me.

– *Big blow?*

– A sudden, devastating answer. Suddenly I realized he decided on our future. He did not let me decide. That's when I got so sick – for a year I could not get over my cold symptoms, asthma attacks and antibiotics. I give everything I have into a relationship. I am not suspicious. I trust. I don't expect the other to play games with me, and he played games with me. He cheated.

– *Describe how you felt during that year.*

– I was very depressed. When he asked, "Why are you still calling me?" I felt like I was slapped.

– *How does it feel to be slapped?*

– It bites into your heart. The same feeling as when I learned I was being cheated on: bursting pressure in the heart. I was asking myself why all my relationships ended so suddenly, so tragically. I was trying to fight it.

> By homeopathic conjecture, this is the story of an insect remedy: strong attraction, busy life and sudden, tragic end. Julia's illness came on when she was cheated on or dumped, when she was not regarded as the "queen and only" anymore. This is how Julia's remedy, Apis, made out of the honeybee, experiences the world. Not only was she cheated on and dumped, she also was not the one who decided. She was not the reigning one. She was not the stronger – she was the weaker – and in that relationship it was clear. That is why she was so devastated when it ended.
>
> Julia emphasizes that one should not play games, should not cheat. She talks about the other party but all these feelings are within her. As such she is sensitive to them; that is why she sees it in others. The way a person sees the world around her describes her inner feeling like a mirror. Often it is much easier to see the nuances in somebody else and we can describe them much better. When somebody tells me a story I listen to all the characters: in what way their attributes are manifestations of the same energy.
>
> So I prescribe a remedy based on this energy pattern, on the fullness of a pattern that has equal and opposite manifestations that play out in all the characters of one's story.

– When my husband hurts me it is the same feeling but it is not that tragic. If I hurt someone I would apologize right away. When

I get hurt I simply don't understand why they hurt me. If I am close to someone I think I cannot hurt their feelings. As much as I understand myself I am able to understand them as well. And within me there are so many contradicting emotions that if I can see that, I can definitely see it in others and not get angry with them. But people have been angry with me, have hurt me, so I am puzzled in those situations. I understand that people react too quickly, too abruptly. They react to a sudden emotion; they get pissed.

> These words further describe how Julia experiences reality as the manifestation of the same energy in herself and in others. She is sensitive to reacting too quickly, abruptly. It does not matter in our case-taking whether she talks about this abruptness in herself or in others. If the energy of abrupt reaction is found in her view of reality, it will be also in the remedy she needs. When she keeps talking about her boyfriends and other people as cheaters, acting too quickly and abruptly, slapping her, or being conceited, these are all qualities that are part of her inner reality. These are all parts of the symptom picture I include in my remedy choice.

– There is no honesty in people. When I was younger I used to lie, but I was so afraid of the consequences that I stopped lying. If the person has something to lose, if his life is at stake, then he becomes more honest. Otherwise, it's just rushing, working every day, no time for anything.

> Through Julia's words, a picture emerges of the specific subkingdom, the insects' world, where her remedy is from. She describes a story of the world of the busy bee that rushes and works all the time. For the queen bee there is devotion from the worker bees and she is jealous of competition, of the next queen. Then there is sudden death. This life cycle is what differentiates this subkingdom from the others.

– *Tell me about your fears.*

– As a kid I had a fear. It, in fact, came back just a couple of days ago: someone would come in to my house, a hairy man coming towards me. A stranger is chasing me. I had to lock the room, it felt so real. When sick, I used to be afraid of that dream. I was petrified if the curtain was moving, I was imagining that someone was coming in. In my dream someone was after me. They invaded my territory.

I also had a recurrent dream. It is a water scene; everything is motionless. There is a big surface of water, very still. There are big black rocks there. The sensation was as if I were levitating. Then there is a fearful, suffocating feeling. Nobody else is there. I don't see myself either. I am all alone, total motionlessness. I feel the strength of the water. I feel the power of the rock. They seemed stronger than my power. That's why it was scary. As if looking at milk or honey. It is gray. Still. It is shiny gray. It is not water; it is thicker, more viscous than water. There is this black rock and I am nearby it. A very unpleasant feeling. Makes me nauseous. It is pulling me towards itself. I cannot get out of it, it is coming closer to me, pulling me closer.

– *Do you remember any physical sensations that came in this dream?*

– Yes. My throat was getting tighter. It is not about drowning in the liquid, just a choking sensation. It was pulling me to itself without words. I was getting closer to it but I never touched it. You couldn't do anything against it. Slowly but surely getting closer, against your will – a timeless feeling, as if you fell into trap and couldn't come back. And you are still not there where you are heading. You are on the road. Nothing bad happened yet.

> This dream is significant. It is an old, recurrent dream that she has had since childhood. The first important aspect of it is that there are two forces: her and a stronger force. She is being pulled by a force bigger than her. This is a sensation in the animal kingdom. Within the animal kingdom we have been seeing characteristics of the insect subkingdom. In this dream

she describes a sensation that is beyond the story line of the dream. It is the vital sensation. It incorporates physical sensations that she has on local levels, such as the choking, the suffocation that she mentioned on several occasions. She gives us a glimpse of how it looks in the realm of her vital sensation. Later we will see how it connects to the remedy she needs.

— On the road?

I ask her about this because she mentioned this phrase earlier when talking about her emotions. Therefore, it could be important.

— Getting closer to something that you do not want, to some tragedy, a negative experience. I am afraid. I do not want to go. Nevertheless, something makes me go closer and closer.

— What is the sensation in this experience?

— The outside circumstances have more power than I do. I do not have the power to say I am not going, nor can I stop that circumstance.

— How do you respond to it?

— I am afraid of the unknown. I have been in situations like this on many occasions, when I was petrified. I was in elementary school when going home from a day trip, and about ten boys walked towards me with flashlights. It was dark. They thought I was a boy, too. They wanted to beat me up. I started running; they were running after me. As I was approaching the building we lived in I was yelling my parents' names, but nobody could hear me. As I entered the building I pressed the button of the elevator. I got lucky: it came before they reached the building, so I could safely go up in the elevator.

— How did you feel in this situation?

— While I was running I was totally scared.

— Describe the scared feeling.

— It is pressure in my heart. I could hear the throbbing in my ears.

— What was the feeling like?

– The feeling was that you do the utmost you can do. You run as fast as you can. Still, you do not how will it end. Once I was in the elevator I was protected; nothing could have happened then. Another incident happened in the neighborhood of my school. A guy in a black suit stopped me. As he opened his jacket I thought I saw knives stuck in there. He offered me candy, dolls and ice cream.

– *Tell me about how you experienced this.*

– I had this feeling that nobody saw it! He was holding my hand tight; I could not escape. My feeling was that even if I screamed for help nobody would be there for me. I knew I had to use my smarts to get out of the situation. I told him, okay, I would go with him, but I needed to get some cigarettes that my parents sent me down for. Surprisingly he let me go and I started running like crazy! After a few weeks I saw him again when I was with a bunch of kids. He kept following us. Later I heard he got beaten up, maybe even died on the side of the road.

Another occasion was when a nine-year-old boy, a few years older than I, came to the bus stop and started talking to me. He asked about my teacher and told me he used to have the same teacher. He behaved very normal, casual. Then he told me he had a package and needed help to deliver it somewhere not far. Yes, of course: he needs help, so I go. We went to his apartment building. When we got in he took off his cloths. He took off my tights. I had to stand with my back to him. I was too small to understand anything but I was sure he would stab me with a knife in my back. He was toying on my legs. I realized that he did not want to kill me, so I got a little calmer. I was thinking: How could I escape? What could I say that would be a convincing story so he would let me go? When he leaned back on the bed I grabbed my bag, rushed out the door and started running down the stairs. It was the same feeling, again. I ran out, down the stairs. I could not open the door. It was too heavy for me to push. He was running after me. I felt I could not get out, oh my god, what's gonna happen... Then, suddenly, someone came home, opened the door and I ran out...

My problem was that I always trusted people. I always believed what people said. Many times similar things happened to me.

— *Tell me more about the feeling of "he would stab me in the back?"*

— I was always afraid of all the bad things another could do to me. How could I free myself from the trap, I always wonder. I am afraid of the chase.

— *What did you feel when you were running?*

— Same feeling in the running away from somebody or when the boy was behind me and I thought he would stab me. I am so petrified that I cannot move, cannot breathe. I am afraid of the unknown.

Another time when I had to flee for freedom was when I was 18, visiting my cousin in a big city. I was at a nightclub. There was a guy whom I really liked. We were dancing, then kissing. Then he suggested that we go for coffee somewhere. Being my first time in the city I had no idea where I was; I just knew that the nightclub was two minutes away from my cousin's house. I did not want to go to another place I did not know. Eventually I agreed to go to a pizza place. Then he said he had to change so he suggested we go to his hotel room. Each time I told him I had to go home, he grew more and more irritated. We drove to his hotel, where he changed. He did not force himself on me but he made some moves while he changed and got completely naked. I did not want to upset him because I had no idea what part of the city we were in. From what I could make out in the dark, I saw a very poor neighborhood. I knew if I asked for help I might get into worse trouble. Even if I ran for help nobody would come. We ended up going to his friends' house. It was the strangest place: his friend was making coffee in the kitchen, then in another room four people were having sex, then in the last room there was this group of Mafia-like figures. A girl was asleep in a corner, supposedly for forty hours because of an ankle injury. They offered me work as a dancer. The guy I was with told them I was his new fiancée. I knew I had to play along; otherwise, I would never get out of there.

— *Tell me about your experience in this situation.*

– There was no way back home. How can I get home? That was the only question on my mind. I told him of course I would marry him. I also told him that my clothes were still in my apartment and insisted on going to get them. At this point I figured he was part of this Mafia. I convinced them to take me home. We drove to my cousin's house and they stopped the car just around the corner. I got out from the car, smiled at them, turned the corner and started to run. I was so scared. I was so disgusted with them. I thought they would not trust me and would come after me. When I got to the door I did not know the combination of the lock. I was pressing all the buttons with shaking hands when someone came home from walking a dog. I got in! As soon as the door closed behind me the terrible feeling was gone.

– *Describe the feeling when the door closed.*

– It felt like safety, that once there they could not reach me.

– *How do you feel while you are running from somebody?*

– I am afraid of being physically hurt.

– *Tell more about that fear.*

– Recently I have been afraid on airplanes. The last two trips I would throw up, I was so afraid. Before that I could not care less. I even used to like it when the weather was a little rough. Or another time I had a car accident. I thought I would die. But neither of these times I felt that terrible scared feeling. I think it is because there was no other person involved in those situations.

> The fear is coming only when there is a "me versus the other" situation. This is a strong indication of the animal kingdom. The situation she is sensitive to is being the victim of an aggressive situation, where others – stronger opponents – are involved. Though she says she is afraid of being physically hurt, her level of fear does not reach the same level when she is in a car crash or afraid on the airplane. She herself makes the connection and says that she is more afraid when another person is involved.

Julia has had the same distinct sensation in her dream, and time and time again it is recurring real-life situations. The sensation is something drawing closer and closer to her. She has to run. It is going to stab her in the back; it is going to hurt her. She is all alone to face this danger, nobody around her to help. This comes through the dream as well as all the situations. Another aspect of this sensation is that she is usually running home, towards safety. This situation narrows the sensation of the animal kingdom into the subkingdom. Based on the type of threat and survival method we are able to identify the subkingdom. As mentioned earlier, these attributes are the hectic, rapid movements, the sexual behavior and the fleeing from danger towards the safety of home. We will see later how all these parts come together.

I ask Julia to tell me about the bulimia.

– I was an overweight kid. It started when I was eight or nine years old. Up to that time I moved a lot, was active, adventurous. But then at school I became an outsider. I wanted to belong to a group. I started putting on weight. They hurt me wherever they could. I felt angry. Why do they hurt me? I did not know why I was different, what made me apart from them. I felt ugly. I did not receive enough encouragement from my parents. They wanted me to achieve in everything. I was not good enough.

When I was fourteen we moved to a big city – it was a completely different world. Rumor had it that all the girls in the city were cool, self-confident, and they all got laid before they turned fifteen. I felt I was just an observer. Things happened to me, passively.

Beside me everybody was controlling my life, and I had bulimia. I started throwing up, making myself throw up. In one year I lost all the weight. I thought I looked good. Boys liked me that way, and I was happy for a few years. Then I wanted to do something for myself, too. My selfishness kicked in. I wanted to do only things I wanted. But I was always afraid that I would make wrong decisions. My tendency was always to blame the others.

> Toward the end of the interview I ask Julia again about the pain in her hands.. She mentions two important things: the pain is stabbing, cutting, as if with knives. It is interesting to note that cutting with knives is a theme that follows her various complaints. It is not only in her physical sensations but also in two assaults where she mentioned how she saw or felt knives. She also adds something about her emotional reactions:

– Now I can cry. I used to hold it all in. I was swallowing all my pain. It all stayed inside.

> The remedy I prescribe is Apis, the homeopathic form of the honey bee. Julia takes a dose of the remedy in 30c potency and her pains subside. When they come back mildly a couple of days later, she repeats the dose and does not need any further doses of the remedy. Two weeks later I get a phone call from her physical therapist. Julia's remarkable recovery prompts her to inquire whether this remedy can be used for other women suffering from pregnancy-induced carpal tunnel syndrome. I explain to her about the individual nature of homeopathic treatment, which she finds fascinating. She is disappointed that she cannot recommend the same remedy to other women but she is happy to learn that she could advise them to look into homeopathy as a promising complementary treatment.
> A few weeks later Julia gives birth to a healthy baby boy!

THE REMEDY SOURCE

Apis is a remedy often prescribed in first aid and acute situations where the condition has similar aspects to a bee sting: puffy, edematous, red swellings that have stinging pains and are ameliorated by cold applications.

In chronic ailments the picture that requires this remedy has more general characteristics of the honeybee. It also has characteristics of its broader groups of the insect subkingdom and animal kingdom, as we saw in Julia's case.

On the local level Julia has edematous swelling of her hands with cutting pains. It makes her move around at night. The swelling has Apis characteristics and the restlessness that the painful swelling creates is a general feature of all insect remedies.

High activity is characteristic of the insect remedies. We see this in Julia's adventurous, active lifestyle, then in her trapped feeling. She also mentions that her decision to get married was a quick one. In fact, she had three situations when it happened to her. Each time there was an element of quick decision based on either attraction to the person or survival instinct. On the most local level she has to move around when in acute pain. These factors all point to the activity level of an insect remedy.

When in danger Julia's first reaction is to run. She runs away from the attacker and runs home to safety. She is getting into a trap that can physically harm her. We can see this energy manifesting in the situation when the queen bee is swarming out and has limited time to get back to the hive in order for the whole hive to survive. Sometimes the queen bee does not make it home.

Bulimia is a disorder that combines the distorted body image, the idea of being attractive and overeating, and leads to a swelling of the body into something larger than its natural state. Again, Apis is the remedy that combines these elements.

Julia talks about not only the swelling in her hands and the physical symptoms of bulimia but also her emotional reaction as not being able to cry. She says everything was held back; she swallowed her tears. This is another point in the case where the same "swelling" energy finds expression on the emotional and physical level.

In Julia's imagination, in fearful situations she had a sensation of being stabbed with a knife, and in reality her carpal tunnel syndrome is expressed as knife-like stabbing pains. Physical and sensational realms are but two manifestations of the same energy.

Choking, or suffocation, is seen throughout the case: in her childhood asthma, the colds she got, the dreams, and the fearful situations. Apis is known to quickly heal swellings of the mucus membranes that cause suffocation. This is a symptom that shows the similarity between the effects of a bee sting and the conditions the remedy is capable of healing.

Her revealing dream describes a pulling force of the milk-like liquid as an outside force that is stronger than she is. As she describes this you can see how the line of her story goes from basic narrative to the emotional level, where she describes her fear. From there she takes us to the level of clearly describing the sensation: the pulling force. She gives us all the details so vividly we can almost touch that milky-white liquid with the black rocks and feel the pulling force. This is the level at which we come closest to the remedy source. This is the realm where the source of the remedy is most intimately revealed. In this case the milky-white liquid can be compared to the royal jelly in which the young queen is being bred.

Royal jelly is a secretion from the head of the bee that aids in the development of immature bees. It is used to feed the young until they develop to their designated rank. If a queen is desired, that specific hatching bee will receive only royal jelly as its food, so that she will become sexually mature and have the fully developed ovaries needed to lay more eggs for the hive. The fears related to the royal jelly can be explained by the fact that a rival virgin queen is often killed in its royal jelly-filled cell by the new queen bee that hatched before her.

One of the characteristic emphases in insect remedies relates to sexuality and reproductivity. Often people needing these remedies have numerous relationships where sexuality is the main driving force. We see this in Julia's emphasis with various men as she describes their relationships. Even as a young girl she entered situations where there was a one-time aspect of the encounter and it was sexual in nature. There is always a quick energy about insect remedies. Just as the insect itself lives a short life, the restless productivity and reproductivity is needed for their survival. We can see the same aspects in Julia's case.

Another relevant factor here emerges from how the hierarchy in the beehive is established around the queen bee. That is why Julia's case not only reveals general insect qualities but also why her idea of being the one and only, the reigning queen, is attractive for her.

When patients talk about their inner sensations, we get glimpses into the inner word of the substance their remedy is derived from. We find points of reference along the way that can help guide us. These are the references that have been uncovered by scientists, scholars of areas of study other than homeopathy: our knowledge of biology, chemistry, of the elements of the periodic table, of the habits and habitats of animals and the qualities of plants. Homeopathic cases are the testimonials of substances translated into human language. They illustrate the inner world of the substance the remedy is derived from. It is a story that fits the blueprint, a story that matches events we know based on empirical or deducted data but fills it up with hard-to-find details. These details have not been available to the human comprehension before, as there have not been tools to measure or observe them. We take the authenticity of this raw data cautiously but when they fit our model and the remedy given based on these details help people to recover from illness, we tend to assume that we are actually acquiring knowledge of the inner structure of these substances.

THE RELEVANCE OF THE BEEHIVE

As described earlier, in the process of finding a suitable remedy for a person we match the energy of the substance with the energy of the person. It is a foreign energy that expresses itself through that person. It is so interwoven into the energy field of the individual that they themselves cannot differentiate between their own energy and that of the foreign energy. This foreign energy is the one that can be matched with a homeopathic remedy. The remedy is the manifestation of that energy. In case of animal remedies, a particular remedy does not manifest only the specific animal that the remedy is made of; it manifests the whole living system that animal lives in. In Julia's case it is not only the specific bee but also the whole hierarchy of the beehive. It is an intricate system of dwelling and functioning. The opposite forces of the structure that keep it working will be seen in the case: the working bee, the queen bee, the old queen bee and the virgin queen that is attacked and killed by the reigning queen. All these forces that keep the hierarchy up manifest in the remedy Apis. These are the opposing energies and forces Julia is talking about and that find expression in her behavior, actions, fears and dreams. Just as a person mirrors her own sensations in other people the remedy reflects the sensations in those in close proximity with it. As we can see in this case the specific characteristic is the quick, "all-or-nothing" quality to it. It is mainly around sexual themes, which brings the insect subkingdom into the picture. Julia's need to be admired and loved comes close to the hierarchy in the beehive, with the queen bee in the center and the worker bees working hard for the survival of the group.

In this case Julia's actions, feelings and sensations describe an image that matches the living structure of bees. As I mentioned earlier, she describes the energies of all the inhabitants of the beehive. This beehive consists of worker bees, which can be male and female, and special breeding chambers for the thousands of future family members. The anatomically identical bees are fed different amounts of royal jelly. Based on the amount each receives, they become different ranks in the hierarchy. For example, queen bees are fed exclusively with royal jelly. They mature to become capable of reproduction.

After the queen bee hatches she leaves the hive for a long flight. Once she is fertilized she has to get back to the hive. She does not have much time for all this, If she does not make it back on time she whole hive is at risk. Sometimes the old queen is still alive when the new queen hatches. In this case a swarm of worker bees surround the queen and kill her or they might take off and find a new home where they starts a new colony. Think about this skit from a queen-bee's life when Julia is telling her stories about running home to safety.

Different aspects of this recount are analogous to Julia's underlying story – not the superficial events but the energy that is beneath it, the forces that find expression through Julia's personality traits and actions. These are all characteristics that make Julia different form other people, just as the beehive is different from other structures of nature. Finding the unique qualities in this unit in nature (i. e., the beehive) and matching them with the energies of Julia is the determining process in deciding on the remedy that will bring a cure. This process makes it possible to find remedies, like Apis in this case, that helped Julia's inner vital force to cure her carpal tunnel syndrome.

A CASE FROM THE EDGE OF THE VALLEY

A Case Taken By Anna Menyhért and Supervised by Ildiko Ran

Even though I have known George for a long time, his initial interview is quite long. Looking back now, and having received Ildiko's insights and advice on the case, I see where I could have recognized the kingdom and the remedy at an earlier point. On the other hand, in the lengthy time it took me to confirm and reconfirm the remedy, it became a beautiful and rounded case. George came very close to naming the exact source of his remedy.

George is sixty years old and suffers from hypertension. He takes daily medication to lower his blood pressure but it still often rises to a peaking degree of 190 or 200. When that happens he gets a headache, feeling pressure in the back of his head, and becomes agitated and nervous. This usually occurs when he cannot decide about an important issue and therefore gets tense.

– I went to renew my driver's license ten years ago. At the health screening I found out I had high blood pressure. I noticed earlier that I had been terribly impatient and some people annoyed me a lot. My doctor told me these were indications of my undiagnosed hypertension. Around the same time my eyesight worsened a lot, probably as a result of bursting blood vessels. When I am tense I cannot even see with glasses. Sometimes I cannot see at all: the letters get blurry.

– *What is the feeling when your blood pressure rises?*

– Stressful, terrible and full of tension. I am less patient; I feel like I cannot handle it anymore. I have the urge to punch something. When my blood pressure is not high I can take it easy; I don't get upset over the same things.

– *How does it feel when you are stressed, full of tension and would punch?*

– Unpleasant, I don't like it. I am helpless. Something is

happening of which I am a part of but I cannot control it. I am inside it and cannot step out.

> This last remark seems to be important, so I ask him about it.

– As a solution my mother used to rearrange furniture in her room every two or three years. I changed jobs every four or five years – not only the specific job but the area of expertise as well. Each time I started doing something completely new. Now for a few years I have had my own company. This is unfortunate because I do not have a chance to go anywhere. I cannot say I will leave this place and look for something new!

– *What is the feeling in leaving?*

– Usually I simply leave. I leave the job and that's it.

– *What is the feeling there?*

– Everything becomes clear and simple. Until I make that decision, though, it is a constant struggle with distressing worries; I feel more and more helpless.

– *Tell me more about the feeling connected to the expression "I am inside it and cannot step out".*

– You can have a dream – which I never had but it is possible – that you stand on the tracks, the train is coming, you should step off. Nothing is holding you there, but still you cannot move. (I have dreams of painful knees and when I wake up it really hurts; I rub it and it goes away.)

– *Something is holding you on the tracks?*

– I never had this feeling; I just gave it to you as an example.

– *I am inside and cannot step out?*

– A situation I cannot change, cannot control. I have to wait out what is going to happen. During these times I eat more, and my sweat glands work harder: sweat is pouring to my eyes, burning, and I will get pimples and blemishes on my head and face. This is also a result of my age; I cannot change too much anymore. I have to suffer the consequences of the wrong choices I have made earlier in my life.

– *I am inside and cannot step out?*

– This is my life. In many ways it is not good, but I cannot do it very differently; I have to live with it.

– *And how is it when you can step out?*

– That is the reason I travel so much. I head to the countryside every weekend. It is a 370-mile round-trip each time. Traveling is the pseudo stepping out. While traveling I feel my life is not relevant, that it is not even my life I am living. My years of growing up were characterized by being on the outside. I was an outsider. I imagined myself sitting on the edge of a big bucket, the edge of a valley, and life was happening down there. Luckily or not I was not in it; I was looking at it from the outside. As a young child I was torn out from the environment I was used to and moved to the country. I grew up in the city and moving to a village was foreign to me. I did not belong to that crowd. I felt an outsider – it did not bother me, though.

Today, stepping out means that I travel around a lot. There is no place I can go to. Everything has narrowed down, closed in. I do not have the time anymore to open new horizons. I have to bear with it; I can tolerate rather than create or influence my reality.

– *How is it that you are not in it but out?*

– I am never in it. It disturbs me when I am in it and cannot change it. Being outside is good because it makes it possible to change things. When I spend the money I sell my possibility to have it for something else. Earlier I did not buy a house because then I would have had to be there constantly.

> The circumstances of George's high blood pressure are becoming clear: the symptoms, the state of mind and his reactions. About all this he talks with the set of two opposites of being inside versus outside. From here on I ask him about these opposites and the powerful image through which he is relating them to me. I phrase my questions based on his own words in order to come closer to the world of his inner sensations.

– *How is it sitting on the edge of the valley?*

– It is a picture of self-pity. It means that I am an outsider. But still, this is better. It is like sitting in front of an aquarium and watching how the fish are swarming in there. I am a fish, too, but I am outside, in a larger aquarium. Since I have been aging I feel I am also in that smaller aquarium.

– *Aquarium?*

– It is transparent. If you are outside in the open air you can see through the glass all that is happening inside the water. You do not need to go in; you can see perfectly well from the outside. If I were inside, I would be closed in, in one place. I prefer going here and there, wherever I wish at the moment. If I were inside I would not see anything. Being an outsider means to be free. For those that are inside, that is the ideal situation, but not for me. By now I have ceased to be an outsider. I got caught in a configuration.

– *Why can't you move freely inside?*

– Because from the infinite possibilities of life situations, one has become mine. Not the infinite possibilities but this certain manifestation. I always thought one had to look forward. If I did something right I did not have to bother with that anymore. If I did something wrong – well, I might need to deal with that. Things interest me only in the planning phase, while I am sketching the outlines. Once it is done I do not want to manage or maintain it; I feel like that is not my business.

> First it seems as if being an outsider means being left out, shunned from the group. But soon it becomes clear that being outside or inside stand for freedom and the loss of freedom. This brings up the relevance of animals, more specifically birds in this case. At this point I ask George a question, hoping it will lead me to the kingdom his remedy is in.

– *What is your relationship with people?*

– Usually I do not let anybody come close to me, and in turn it disturbs me when others want to let me get close to them. I like to be an outsider. If I meet people I dislike, I try to excuse myself from their friendship.

In this answer we see a variation of the same pair of opposites: the counterpart of "outside" now becomes "close to me." From here on I narrow it down to the animal kingdom as I see that as the most prominent possibility. At this point I am not sure if my assessment is correct, but later Ildiko points out to me that whenever I ask George to describe the outside and inside, he goes deeper and tries to describe it from a different angle. More and more ideas enter the story that might seem out of place but already, after my second question, George is talking about his inner experience of the "inside–outside" polarity.

– Have you been competitive at your jobs?
– I have always been very competitive. It stems from my childhood when the community did not accept me and I had to confront them, fight them. I either prevailed or got overpowered.

The animal kingdom is clear now: winning or losing is at stake in a fight.

– To fight?
– It was not out of my own will. They were teasing me for my name and for not being familiar with the ways of village life. One day they started hurling rocks at me. I stopped, faced them and told them to throw the rocks from that tree; they couldn't get me anyway. Of course I picked a tree that was far away. They were hurling the rocks and I was just standing there. There were fights like this. In school there were no fights since I was the smartest kid in the village.

– Is there anything that is humiliating for you?
– When I am forced to do something I do not want to do. I recall an unpleasant situation, which haunted me for years: it is a memory of being ashamed because I got frightened, panicked – I lost control over myself. Back then I decided it would never happen to me again. I was seventeen; the eighteen-year-olds were being drafted into the army. They had their last night out when one of the drunken boys called to me: "Hey, what's up kid?" I

said, "Call me a kid and I will slap you!" Then his pal came and I told him off the same way. They pulled knives out of their pockets. I said, "Catch me if you can!" and ran off. As I was running, suddenly two other guys approached from the sides. It was dark. I was caught by surprise: there were four of them and they cornered me. I got scared. I was afraid they would beat me up. Instead they lectured me. I completely forgot that one of the rules of the village was that many kids were not supposed to gang up on one. In this case I should have just said, "Hey, I am outnumbered" and that would be the end of that. I was so scared I forgot to think; I forgot what I was supposed to say.

– *What was the worst part of that experience?*

– How could I have lost my control over my mind? I should have known better. I should have known that they couldn't beat me up because of the village ethics. I decided that I would never lose self-control again, whatever happened to me.

– *What happens if you lose self-control?*

– I am defenseless against outside forces. I cannot comprehend what happens to me: sheer terror. Like a wave of panic, an out-of-body experience: now I am finished, I will die. Like drowning. I experienced that once – I could not swim and I was in deep water. Ever since I have had an aversion to water even though I am a good swimmer.

– *What is the out-of-body experience like?*

– Losing self-awareness or self-control. My whole life, that was the only incident when I lost the clarity of seeing the situation from the outside and myself in it.

> The way George experiences these situations – as conflicts – points to the animal kingdom: he failed himself against his own mind; he is defenseless to outside circumstances. His choice of words brings up the main polarity again: outside is embedded in the meaning of "out-of-body." For him an out-of-body experience brings about the inability to see himself and the situation from the outside. He cannot

step out from inside of the situation. It is an interesting twist on this sensation. Out-of-body becomes inside, which is the negative polarity of his sensation. He loses self-control, he becomes defenseless, he feels he is drowning.

– *In the situation when the boys came at you with pocketknives, from the sides, and you were outnumbered, you lost control, you came to an out-of-body experience that felt like drowning, panic, sheer terror?*

– At that time there was no drowning. I mentioned it as that can evoke a similar sensation for someone who cannot swim and is pushed into the deep water. He might start swimming, thinking he can reach the bottom. But once past the four-foot-deep end of the pool – this happened to me as a teenager – I thought I could rest for a moment, but when reaching for the bottom of the pool it was not there. I swam quite well for a few yards but this feeling of not reaching the bottom made me panic. I started flailing my arms, was in a shock, out of my body. In this state of mind you don't even notice if you are again in the shallow water and your feet could reach the bottom.

– *What is this shocked state like, the out of body and flailing?*

– I never thought about it. Being shocked is quite a common concept. But it felt like when you prick a balloon. I was running like a conceited idiot, thinking nobody could beat me because just a week before that I had won the school's 400-yard race. At that moment my whole reality collapsed: out of the nowhere three other guys blocked me. My world turned upside down. Like when you prick the balloon and it bursts. A total collapse. Nullified.

> Here George starts gesturing with his hands, which until now has not happened. It is obvious that he is getting closer to his core sensation. He is moving his arms up and when he talks about plummeting he drops them in his lap.

– It is the feeling of plummeting from the total ruling down to zero. The contrast is too big. Nowadays, if I get overly excited my blood pressure rises, my head becomes hot. I assume it is related to the rigidity of the blood vessels. If I recall it correctly, this heat came over me back then, too. But I am not sure about it.

> George talks about symptoms that accompany his chief complaint – the high blood pressure – but also appear in other situations: feeling the heat-wave, a general sensation of heat that comes along with the plunging, becoming zero and being pricked.

– *Feeling of zero, balloon is being pricked?*
– I had a mini-experience of it a few days ago playing chess on the Internet. I was in the leading position when I took a step and realized what a terrible mistake it was: I sacrificed my queen, left her completely defenseless. She was easily taken and I lost the game. Then this heat wave suddenly flooded me. The contrast was big. I thought I would win the game and then suddenly I realized that I lost it.
– *And you felt the heat flooding you?*
– Yes, it is caused by contraction of the blood vessels.
– *Talk more about the balloon that is pricked, the feeling of zero, shocked state, the out of body and drowning sensations, flailing and the heat wave.*
– This is obviously a mildly shocked state, when one realizes that he has done something dumb. Once something similar happened at work. I was the program manager and coordinator for a project that involved several people. The project almost completely failed because I lost sight of an important detail. When I realized this I felt like I was not going to survive. It lasted about twenty minutes. How could I be so dumb? I had this same feeling, the sensation of heat. It is like when you are walking in the woods and suddenly you fall into a dark pit, unexpectedly falling down in the darkness.
– *Have you had the same sensation at any other time? In physical complaints or dreams?*
– Last time when my blood pressure rose to 185, I had a terrible headache. It was a result of having to face some people on a project and tell them all the work might needed to be canceled.

That night my daily chores came in my dream in very tangible, realistic forms: it was like a mill, a grinder. I was in the throat of that grinder in a trapped position. My chores are in there but cannot go through the grinder. They are just turning, turning, turning in there. One keeps popping out; I cannot force it through the grinder. It comes back up again and again. It does not get ground, cannot stay in there, but keeps popping back up. The problem cannot be resolved. It might be related to that the previous week I was grinding apples and an awful lot of apples indeed kept popping up. The problem cannot be solved. It cannot get into that phase when it could be solved in some way.

– *Turns, turns, pops out?*

– When it pops out it is like failure, shock, disappointment. When you serve in Ping-Pong and the third time it ends in the net.

– *How does it feel?*

– Helplessness. That I am serving and serving and it always gets in the net.

> I ask him to once again show the gesture he used when talking about the popping out and describe it a little more.

– In the grinder there are two cylinders rotating, and on them there are spikes and thorns. In a funnel there is the stuff to be ground and it is flowing down towards the opening between the cylinders. There it gets stuck, presses through and drops out. If the spikes cannot grab into the apple pieces they jump up and pop out. This we can prevent by cutting up the apple.

– *What is the popping out like?*

– Maybe my choice of this synonym is appropriate because one is expecting to be fulfilled and realized and when he feels very close to the finish line, feeling he got it, the whole thing falls apart, collapses. A bummer, being nullified – but this is not the best word to describe it.

– *Disappear, blow up, nullified?*

– Suspenseful anticipation – you almost got it and then suddenly it escapes you; you do not have it.

– Do not have it?

– It is a sudden loss of energy. You feel like you have got it and suddenly you do not. Then you feel blank, the end of all. Back to zero. It lasts only for a short time. So you try again. You again feel like you are getting there, and then, puff, suddenly you are back to zero; as a result of all your straining you are back down again. Then you climb up to the highest point just to fall back again.

– Can you connect the…

– The grinder with the pit? That is perishing, too. Pops out – perishes. The pricked balloon perishes, too. In the pit it is crashing – perishes.

Regarding the grinder in the dream, some things got mixed up, as if I were the problem and that stuff that needed to be ground as well. I could not go through the narrow opening. I felt I needed to get through it somehow, to press myself through it, but I couldn't do it.

– What was that like?

– Depressing, I guess, to get stuck. Finally I think it is going and then it does not. As if I were trying to get out of a cave and I don't succeed; I always slip back. The whole thing seems hopeless.

> As George is talking about his dream he keeps gesturing with his hands, using variations of the same basic movement. When he is talking about the grinder he is rolling his fists around. When talking about the apple popping out, he opens his hands and with some momentum he tosses them upwards. When talking about the crashing diving, he drops his arms. Then he is climbing upwards with his arms, reaches for something, then drops them again. He is reaching forward and up with hands in tight fists. Then, when talking about hopelessness, his hands drop in his lap. People who need animal remedies often speak the language of the source: they tell stories or recount their dreams that are characteristic of the animal's life

circumstances, either short snapshots or longer, more multifaceted accounts of the animal's daily life. Often the homeopath hears this underlying story but still cannot identify the remedy, as the exact level or placement of the story is not established in the case. In George's dream the grinder belongs to the human world and his daily experiences but the sensations he describes his experience with indicate the animal kingdom. We can see this in his choice of words and gestures: at first he describes the apple pieces being pressed down and popping up, but soon he describes these motions as active "climbing up" and "'falling down."

I can tell that this dream is really important to George. These images are almost jumping in my face, but I am not sure what they are telling me. So I decide to change the subject, hoping that arriving at his core sensation from a different direction will shed light on this dream as well.

– *How do you react to pain?*

– I don't freak out. I do not tend to scream and whine. I used to be afraid of pain – not the pain itself but rather what it was an indication of. I think fear of pain gets mixed up with fear of death and becomes replaced by it. I assume it is the case with everybody but I know for sure it is the case with me. When you know you will not die from the cause of the pain or will not get any major defect from it – will not go blind, for example – one can endure it easily. It hurts but it will go away.

Once, around the time I was ten, I had an infected thumb, which the doctor cut open without any anesthetics. I could tolerate it well as he cut into the flesh and did not feel any pain, but I felt as if suddenly I flew upwards, that I was soaring. I lost consciousness and when I woke up I was sitting, with my thumb bandaged. I had a similar soaring experience a few years prior to that when, out of curiosity, I broke open an old, rusty tube with an axe. It had pure nicotine in it – a form of undiluted pesticide – which squirted in my face and eyes. As I was regaining consciousness a few minutes later, I saw some dead chickens around me lying on the ground. Some drops from the tube sprayed into their drinking water.

– *When the doctor cut your thumb? It was as if you flew up, soared?*

– That did not hurt. He told me to sit down because it would hurt and I told him it was fine, he could cut. He agreed and put it there.

He gestures a lance with his fingers.

All I felt was him touching it, then for a split second some burning heat. The next thing I knew I was sitting in an armchair, my hand bandaged, and the doctor was slapping my face in an attempt to wake me up.

– *And the flying up, soaring sensation?*

– The lance touched it, then the burning sensation and then this, this...

> Here George cannot explain the sensation with words: he starts using the same gesture he used when talking about the apples. The only difference now is that he is moving his arms in larger circles and he follows the circles with his upper body and head, too. I ask him to show these movements once again and to describe them more.

– Lightheadedness. As if I flew up or got woozy. Like when you get dizzy on a merry-go-round. Like giddiness or heat wave. Your body is flooded with heat, mild giddiness, hot head; the whole body gets hot and then in a few minutes it is all gone.

> A new word appears: flying. As we continue the interview, George starts using more and more expressions that make it clear he needs a remedy from the animal kingdom. As he adds the notions of flying and soaring, he starts hinting the bird subkingdom.
>
> The sensation of flying and soaring is important

because he experiences it in connection with feeling hot, which in turn is one of the main components of his specific way of experiencing his chief complaint: high blood pressure.

As George is putting his sensations into words when answering more and more questions, we can see how his words describe his inner sensation and his remedy in a more specific way. Each answer includes the inner knowledge of the level of sensation that he covered earlier, and each time he takes it one step further. That is why each time we seem to hit a dead end, I return to the same questions that he had answered previously.

– Tell me what is pleasant for you. How do you experience pleasant sensations?

– I love driving fast.

– Why?

– I enjoy speed. As a kid I loved sledding. There I loved the speed, too. I loved how fast I was going down the hill.

– What was the feeling like?

– If I have to name it, I would say it is getting from one point to the other very fast. You are there but not there anymore.

– Anything else about it?

– Flying. I loved riding my bike, too. It is a good feeling.

– Why did you have to fight when the kids were teasing you in school?

– What do you mean why I had to fight?

– Not everybody would fight in a situation like this.

– I could never bear to be defeated, if someone beat me in anything.

– Why?

– I don't know. I was born this way.

– What is the feeling like when you are defeated?

– It is not the right way to say it. It's not that I cannot bear to be defeated, because in something I will be defeated for sure. But I cannot bear not solving things I could solve in principle.

– Why do you need to fight?

– I cannot give up anything.

– *Like what?*

– Anything I am serious about.

– *Say more about that.*

– Let's stay with the example of the kids hurling rocks at me. More or less I could see through those kids. I had a good understanding – and still think I was right – of their motivations. They could not see through me. And because I was superior in this respect I just could not imagine that I could be anything less than superior in other areas of life.

– *Why?*

– Just because. I obviously do not go to a territory where I am in an inferior position. Once I decide to enter a territory, if I risk it, then I must be the winning one.

– *Why?*

– Because that's who I am. I was born this way. Later in my life it has been the same way: if I came to any new environment after a few days of adjusting and getting a hang of things, I became the leader somehow. I could not stop myself. Situations where there was no chance for this I would avoid from afar. Maybe that's how I expressed defiance. I was five years old when from a loving, caring environment I dropped into a harsh, rejecting place. The villagers let us know that we were not welcome. We were town folks, not respectable from their point of view. The young lads in the village voiced their displeasure by snarling obscene remarks at my mother. This kind of attitude that surrounds you and seeps into you can bring about only hatred and resistance. It brought about a feeling, that "Hey, you bastards, I will return this favor to you."

– *How would you call it in other words?*

– If one meets hostility or aggression – because it is aggression – there are two possibilities. One is that he is the weaker one and collapses. The other is that he is the stronger one and hits back. In my case that's what happened. I was the stronger and I hit back. I did not beat them up but I told them they could not reach me: you can rave up a storm but will not get me with the damn rocks. They never got me, never, even though there were five of them.

– *What is this feeling like?*

– Victory.

– *What is that like?*

– You become light, like when you drive fast.

– *Victory, light? They cannot reach you?*

– I don't know.

> Sensations of the animal kingdom and more specifically the bird subkingdom are emerging here: fight, where being the weaker or the stronger is at stake. The winner senses victory that is accompanied by lightness. We are coming closer to a certain group of birds: speeding in the car is like flying, fainting like soaring. He usually becomes the leader of a group whereas situations where he cannot achieve he avoids from afar. Now what's left is for George to tell me which specific bird he needs.

– *What about the pain, where is the fear of pain in these situations?*

– It is not the fear; it is the horror of mortal fear. When I think of pain specifically, if for example someone says they were slashed in the thigh with a knife, or if I know I would get an injection, I get a crawling sensation in my shin. This is not fear; it is a horrible feeling.

> He points at his shinbone, pulling his hand upward from down, as if he is detaching, peeling off something from there.
>
> At this point I am thinking of a bird that eats the flesh off the bones of its prey – a raptor. It is important that his sensation of the pain is specific to cut, stabbed wounds. So I keep asking further about this specifically. After a while I do not need to ask because George keeps talking on his own, emphasizing his words with gestures.

– As if someone pulled out the bone from my shin, a horrible feeling. As if someone were nibbling on my bone, but only my shinbone. Sawing my shinbone, sharp teeth digging into it, as if a rat were gnawing at it.

This is exactly the feeling I get when I imagine someone else's pain. When I hear that someone was stabbed in the belly or stepped on a nail, I feel as if the bone was gone from my leg. Fuzzy, gnawing sensation, as if my legs were about to disappear and I collapsed. As if my legs turned into jelly, the firmness vanished from it. A shinbone specific shudder.

– *What you are saying is that the pain is caused by an outside force?*

– Yes. There are two types of pain. One is caused by someone either on purpose or by chance. You get slashed by a sword or step on a nail. If I think about internal pains, like I have a stomachache, a headache – these do not bring about such a sensation. Only intrusion, destruction does. Internal pain is almost natural.

– *Do you get this sensation only in the case of cut and puncture wounds?*

– Yes. This is the type of pain caused by a firm object. Scalding with hot water is not like this. It needs to be destruction caused by a firm object: knife, needle, axe, scythe, anything that cuts and causes damage, like a doctor's lance.

– *What is the feeling like when you cut your finger?*

– While I am cutting I don't get this sensation. I do not feel it then. it is not painful because it happens so fast – I notice it later on. You do not have the time to imagine it happen. It comes only if a pocketknife, scissors or needle pierces in there. I cannot feel the piercing itself because it happens so fast. I sense it a few moments later, when I see it bleeding.

> All this confirms the raptor bird. George feels the dread of pain only if a sharp-piercing object causes the wound: that's how the raptor bird wounds its prey.

– *When you get an injection what are your sensations?*

– Usually I fear they would pierce the periosteum. Before the shot I have this eerie sensation in the shinbone so usually I ask them to give it in the upper arm where the bone is deeper.

– *If they pierce the periosteum?*

– That's awful: the needle is scraping, poking at the bone. Edgar
Allan Poe has a short story *(The Pit and the Pendulum)* in which
rats are chewing a rope away as the pendulum descends. It is
coming closer and closer, down towards you, and you imagine
how the knife is coming closer, how it will soon slash into your
flesh. That's how I feel it in my shinbone.

> As George is talking about the pendulum he is swaying
> his arms: first just one finger, then his whole hand
> with stretched-out palm, lowering his arms. It looked
> like a large bird swaying from side to side before crash-
> diving on its prey. As he talks about the pendulum
> from Poe's short story and then brings up memories
> of a church bell he uses words to describe this large
> bird. The pendulum comes to life as a bird: a large,
> ready-to-attack predator that flies hissing through the
> air, whooshing above the heads of those standing
> beneath, gliding, slithering, then diving down fast and
> precise as a bullet. At the end of the rope in the short
> story there is a curved knife attached – like the hooked
> beak of raptor birds.

– The hero of the short story is in jail, in a pit, a kind of hopper
underneath the ground. They strap him to the table. In the cupola
the pendulum is swinging, with the sharp knife hanging at the
end of the rope. With each swing the pendulum lowers an inch
and evidently at some point it will reach the table, slicing the
man. But he uses some rats to chew the ropes that tie him down
and manages to roll off the table at the last minute. In the story
the swinging of the ever-lowering pendulum is described in
painstaking detail, affecting all our senses. As a teenager I was
reading it, imagining the hissing pendulum moving through the
air. I was appropriately shuddering.
Once in Moscow I saw a pendulum that was designed to swing in
sync with the rotation of the globe. As it was turning along it was
flying over different parts of the world map. You are standing
there and can hear how the pendulum is ripping through the air.

As it is swaying it stops at the out-most points. It picks up speed until it reaches the center and then slows down again. It needs to defeat the resistance of the air, thus continuously losing its speed.
– *Flying?*
– A large, jar-like heavy object with a dart at the tip is hanging on a long, thin chain. If the large heavy object were not there I would say it swings, but the large object gives a feeling of free flight. Buzzing above your head as you are looking up. If you are at the right angle you can see both end points of its trajectory and it seems like it is swinging. If you are standing right underneath, it suddenly appears from the dim background. It is a huge object dashing at you, zooming by, flying and sweeping away. It does not even seem like a pendulum but rather some other grim object that speeds by at the level of your eyes. It cuts through the air, hissing as it crash-dives like a bomb. As it dives the squawk gets louder, which is caused by the splitting-speed. You can hear that whistle-like sound. A dreadful experience to stand under that pendulum and imagine the pendulum falls off the chain and whoosh – does not stop all the way to St. Petersburg.
– *Squawk?*
– Grazing sound like the sound of wind. The fierce wind out in the woods. A totally captivating experience.
– *Captivating?*
– It makes you captive, spell-bound. Does not let you go free. It is like watching the pendulum: you cannot stop following it with your eyes. I wanted to stay there but I forced myself to leave.

> George has not realized it yet, but he is talking about a bird in picturing his own sensations in the flight of the pendulum, which is his own flight-sensation. Soon he realizes what he is really talking about: what is captivating in his own life, how it is related to his chief complaint: high blood pressure.

– *Let's go back to the feeling of victory which is light like the speeding in the car.*

– Interestingly enough, I never wanted to be a paratrooper, even though there I could really live this experience. Maybe because when I was a young boy there was another kid who went to do some parachute jumps and his parachute did not open so he died. They collected him in pieces. After that it was not a popular sport in our village.

I like speed because of the feeling that I can be here and there at the same time.

– *Can you speak more about this?*

– The other ingredient needed for the experience of speed is the sound of it. When I drive a quiet car I enjoy it less, as some element is missing. If I roll the window down or open the sunroof, then the speed experience is perfect. I need the hissing of the wind to feel the experience with all my senses and to acknowledge with my mind, too that I am flying with an extreme speed.

> George swings both his arms forward, showing the fast flying.

– *You are flying?*

– I think danger is not included in this experience, even though I know that any time I could crash into something and if there were any problem I would die instantly, especially because I am going 100 miles per hour on a country road. At several occasions I saw car wrecks that had crashed into deer or boars at night. I have killed wild hares before.

> As he mentions the hare, George starts circling with his index finger. This is a frequently used gesture in people who need the remedy made of falcon.

– I know it can happen any time but the main feeling is not that I am risking something but the sheer joy of flying.

> He again throws both of his arms forward.

– *Tell me how it is to fly!*

– I cannot say besides that it is great. You are light, weightless, not tied down.

– *Tied down? Is there any time when you feel tied down?*
– When I play chess and cannot stop it. The feeling then is as if I was tied, glued to the chair or to the screen. I keep trying to stop it but somehow I cannot. It feels like helplessness: I have decided fifty times that that's it, this was the last one, I've had enough. My blood pressure keeps rising, and I say it does not matter anymore, and then that's it, I am done. But by that time I notice that I started yet another game.

> When he says "that's it," he gestures a cutting motion with his finger, exactly the same way he gestured the doctor cutting his infected finger. Finishing with the "tied down" feeling, that's what this gesture signifies. At the doctor, dizziness – flying up – followed the cutting.

– *How are the not being tied down, the fast flying and glued there related?*
– They are related. Being glued there means that I am stuck to that problem: that is the polar opposite of flying – the fast driving. I am stuck even though I decided a long time ago that I would stop doing that and I keep noticing myself still doing the same thing.

> When he mentions the word flying he throws his arms forward, then drops them down. Then, as he says stuck, he closes his hands into fists and pulls them up and down, like a bird flapping fast and then trying to get out of a bond.

– *Do you have any physical sensations connected to this?*
– I hear hissing in my ears, like the sound of wind. This is the elevated blood pressure when I am tense. I can hear the blood pulsating through my veins. It is probably coming from the calcified discs that resonate to the pulsation of the blood. By the way, it also happened when I was a kid, especially when I could not fall asleep. I was just lying in bed in silence, my head and ears pressed into the pillow. I could hear, just like now, the quiet rushing of blood. I remember this as a pleasant sensation: listening to this inner sound, I could remove myself from my

surroundings, actually floating, levitating above the room. And in this situation all the little noises of the room – crackling furniture or scurrying of the mice – sounded like explosions and brought me back to reality.

– *What about flying? Describe the physical sensation.*

– Bursting breast.

   He opens his arms excitedly.

– Like when you are listening to beautiful classical music, like the *Egmont Overture* or *The Ride of the Walkurs*. Filled with air, expanding, floating. It brings tension, but it is pleasant tension, like speed.

– *And the floating?*

– Let me correct that: the floating is not speed. Floating is stationary. Jellyfish float. I become distant, rise up, rise above, as if I were far above it all, high up, as if I were not down here.

– *Rise up?*

– Nothing matters anymore. Most things lose their significance. You hear the rushing of blood and from this constant noise – it must be self-hypnosis – you not really float but you become distant from your own reality. Then the bed creaks and you suddenly drop back down.

– *What is the feeling?*

– Very good feeling. It is like… Bach's *Pastorale;* that music is like that. You reach infinite distance. Like when you go up on a high mountain, but not to the snowy peaks, just under the snow-barrier. You rise up, ascend from the ground. Mountains in Transylvania are like that. There are wide, spacious valleys stretched below. As if you came to a void, far from everything. Or you go up to the fort of Fuzer and can see everything below from there. When I first went to the fort of Arva I thought about the people who used to live here; they must have seen the world from a very different perspective. You can understand how their way of thinking was different from their peasants. Those who see the world from such an elevation will not be bothered by small, trivial things. It is of course not the actual reality but that's how I imagined it then, that the ways of the everyday world down below were not relevant to me and it was good because that world was full of problems.

In this last stretch George is telling me everything I want to hear, and even more, his words are emphasized by hand gestures. When he is talking about rising above, he is lifting his arms above his head, palms facing down, making small "fluttering" motions. When talking about the valley below he is waving his arms around his waist making small, clicking motions with his fingers to illustrate the small, trivial things. Everything matches now: his sensation of filling up with air and expressing it with musical examples are characteristics of bird remedies. The opposite of this inflation could have been the crashing, nose-diving, nullification – when the balloon is pricked. In the last image he revisits the first one: sitting outside in the edge of the valley. The physical attributes are present as well – rushing of blood, which when George is not able to rise above the trivial problems of everyday life, when he feels like he is glued to the chair, comes to expression in the rising blood pressure.

After taking the remedy Falco peregrinus (about which you can read more in the next case) in the 30c potency, George's tension vanishes, his optimism returns. He still takes his medication for hypertension, but whereas earlier it did not prevent the blood pressure rising to 185 degrees, with the remedy these incidents happen less frequently. So he occasionally takes single doses of the remedy while steadily improving.

HOMEOPATHIC INTERVIEWING OF CHILDREN

Most of the cases we have studied are of adults that can articulate their inner sensations well and who understand questions aimed at their emotions and sensations, questions that require a degree of maturity. Homeopathy also is a useful treatment modality for children, but the interviewing style is different. Often we see the parents separately from the child and ask them to describe their child: their usual reactions and characteristics that make them different from their siblings or other children.

Interviewing adults follows a pattern that is more or less predictable. In cases of children some special rules apply. Children often cannot verbalize their state of mind to the point adults can. However, they have a great advantage over adults: they express, they live their sensations. If we ask and listen, they will share with us their inner experience on a truly authentic level.

Children often do not want to be told what to do, or how to do it. If we ask them specific questions it is easy to miss the essence. If we allow them to pick the topic of their choice, however, we will hear the essence in each sentence! When a goal-oriented task needs to be completed, such as an interview with a specific goal in mind, it can be challenging to channel children's energy in the right direction. But on a journey into the child's inner feelings the best and shortest way is the seemingly winding road they are taking. It is like walking with them to the park and noticing how they keep climbing each stair, railing and wall. If we follow them on those "side" steps we will understand their experience before reaching the park. The same happens in the interviewing process. We listen to what they are eager to talk about and follow the path they lay out.

Most children live in the realm of their imagination so that is where this path usually takes us. Talking about their favorite activities, movies, sports – it will all lead us to the same inner experience.

There are babies who do not yet talk and there are adolescents who have stopped talking. There are talkative children, those that make up stories and those that have trouble communicating. We need to find what works with each age group, with each specific child, depending on his or her ability level and communication skills. Working with children is challenging in its own way, but it is also greatly satisfying. One of the most important aspects of this work is to observe the child. In my own practice, while I listen to the words of the parents I keep observing the child. It is fascinating how many ways children behave in the office. Some sit on their mother's lap; some keep fidgeting, pulling out books, magazines and pens; some keep annoying their parents or siblings; some quietly draw or build with toys. Most children are eager to talk; I just have to find the key to their chatterbox.

Valuable information comes with spontaneous behavior. Children's misbehavior can be the most useful information we gather during the interview. Parents might try to intervene and stop the misbehavior or their chattering answers to my questions. When that happens, I gently remind them that it is in the child's best interest right now to talk that nonsense or to misbehave.

Homeopaths work in their own unique way and schedule their visits accordingly. In my practice most children come in after I have met with their parent for an initial visit. This way I get the "story" along with mental and emotional concerns that are easier to discuss without the child being present. At the subsequent visit, when the child comes in, I can listen to the inner story, the way the child experiences it, and ask specific questions regarding their friends, dreams and favorite activities. The unfolding case often defies the picture I was getting from the parent!

Let's look at a case of a seven-year-old girl. I will call her Lucy.

A Case of a Seven-Year-Old Girl with Chronic Eczema

Lucy is the second of four children in a loving family.
Both parents are artists and the children are blessed
with great talents and a love of nature. First I talk to
the mother without Lucy being present:

– Lucy was very serious as an infant. I think the main difference
between her and her siblings was that it was so difficult to get
her to smile. Ever since, she has been conscientious. She worries
all the time: "Dad, the speed limit is 45! Mom, there is no parking
sign."

She is deeply concerned with rules. She wants to abide by them
and wants others do the same. She weighs the consequences;
she predicts and is concerned about what is going to happen.
On the other hand she can incorporate any criticism. She does
not get easily upset. She is rebellious, not trying to please others.
She can comfort herself and has self-confidence. She knows
exactly what she wants. For example, she would say something
like "I want to eat a juicy thing." She is not just asking for a
snack; she is more specific than that. She knows what her body
needs and makes sure she gets it.

She has had eczema on and off since she was an infant. At the
age of four it got a lot worse. She would get an attack and it
would spread all over her body. The first bad attack came after a
vacation in Maine, on a lake.

– *How does Lucy react to the eczema?*

– She always denied her eczema. She rebelled against it, does
not want to deal with it. She does not like to be pitied or have
someone feel sorry for her. She is difficult to hug, to cuddle. She
is prickly!

Even though people come to see a homeopath with
specific complaints, they often start telling their story

with a seemingly random subject. It is very important that we follow this lead and later on inquire about the chief complaint. Lucy's mother is telling me very important characteristic traits about her daughter, which might have not come up if we started talking about the eczema right away. Once we get to the eczema she describes it in general details, the way she would in a doctor's office. I need to ask her to be more specific. In homeopathy the person's reaction to their ills has the most value in finding a healing remedy for them. The technique is to follow the flow, follow the words that describe the inner sensation. There are words that people use to describe specific complaints. We, homeopaths listen to the words that are not the common ones used in a typical conversation. So when Lucy's mother says prickly, it has the most weight for me in her description because it is the most unusual word.

– *Please describe that prickly.*

– She will pull in or make a face. She does not want affection. But I think it is more a reaction to the physical embrace. She enjoys being in the family; it is important for her. She shows affection to us and to her siblings. The actual physical affection – hugs and cuddling – seem to be constraining for her. I have an image of her that she wants to run free. She is rebellious, has the bravado about her. But it does not mean she does not need the affection.

In her answer to my question about a simple word she describes a child who is reacting to physical contact in a certain way. She describes Lucy as someone who loves freedom and does not like constraints. In her answer there seems to be emphasis on the interaction between Lucy and her siblings or parents. It is not a reaction to a sensation; the mother is not listing sensations related to prickly but rather tells about actions and Lucy's reactions. This emphasis is characteristic of the animal kingdom and the reference to freedom brings the bird

realm to mind. It is too early to narrow it down to one
realm but we can see some clues in the story.

When we talk about Lucy's interests, her mom tells
me that she loves books, loves reading. She does not
read a book cover to cover, though. She starts reading,
then stops and makes up the end of the story herself!
She fills the stories in her mind. She is very imaginative,
using the pieces to make her own original stories.

– *What are the main themes of her originals?*

– She loves animals, loves them with passion. She not only writes
fiction about them but also reads books like animal encyclopedias;
she knows a great deal of facts about animals.

– *Tell me more about her relationship with animals.*

– She has a way with animals and feels strongly about them. She
is not afraid of any animals.

Lucy's mother keeps making references to Lucy's love
for animals. We often see it in people who need
remedies of the animal kingdom.

– She stays cool-headed with people, too. She is not bossy but
negotiates. She can bring people along. For her there is no
conflict, no obstacle. She works it through. She is rebellious and
at the same time conscientious. It is important for her not to do
anything wrong. In school she is concerned with things you are
supposed to do or not supposed to do. On the other hand, she
is messy: she throws her clothes and books on the floor; she is
untucked, not worried about how she looks. Things that are not
important to her, she won't care about. But she is very serious
not to cross the street.

Another problem is that she has accidents because she does not
want to go to the bathroom. She wants to be free to continue
what she is doing but then she cannot hold it anymore. I see the
same in her refusing to acknowledge her skin problem. She does
not want anything to be wrong with her because she perceives it
as something that makes her stay back. She experiences her
differences with her brother, who is two years older than her, as

painful. In her mind she needs to excel, to surpass her brother. It is devastating for her when he wins in something, when he excels in something more than she does. So she does not want her skin to be an issue because it might hold her back. It is not a problem for her. She does not want people to feel sorry for her. She resists that, brushes it off. If we talk about her eczema she changes the subject.

> This short passage confirms the homeopathic view of the animal kingdom. Lucy seems to be rather competitive. It is important for her not to lose. The main problem for her with her eczema is that it stops her from doing things freely, from getting ahead. In her reality the problem is not the itchiness or the look of her skin (as it is for many other eczema sufferers). For her it is the staying behind, the losing in the competition that matters. Her eczema is the means by which her body is keeping her back.
>
> This is what we elicit by this type of questioning, and this is the direction I will head during the interview. I have to find Lucy's individual reaction to her complaints, and the essence of the healing remedy will be found there. So far I have seen part of the picture, but I have to go further and deeper to see how competition affects her. So far I have heard about Lucy's need for freedom, which in homeopathy mostly comes across in the bird subkingdom. Within the bird subkingdom we have several remedies with their own characteristic symptoms. With careful inquiring I will narrow that down to the most suitable remedy.

– Lucy is a seeker of ecstatic experiences. She loves to be taken somewhere else. Whenever she has the possibility she loves rolling down a hill. She wants to become dizzy. It is like spinning. She is seeking to go to the edge, bursting out.

– *Please describe this experience when she gets to this state.*

> This is an important part of the interview because

this is where energy is showing in its purest form.
This is the part where we can get a glimpse of Lucy's
inner experience.

– It is an intoxicating place. She becomes giddy, radiant! She is
in bliss. She could not be happier… The only other time I have
seen her in this state is when she is with animals. There is some
disheveledness about her. Her energy focuses and she lights up,
glowing: her eyes are bright, her skin is beautiful. It goes on and
off all of a sudden.

There is intensity in her. She is alive and ecstatic. The whole
world disappears. She is a mess, but glowing!

This kind of experience is characteristic of a few groups
of remedies. One of these groups is the bird group.

– She is extremely long and limber. She is good at gymnastics,
has a beautiful headstand and cartwheel. She loves spinning.
There are these two polarities in her: she loves the physical activity
– the running, spinning, exploring – but she also has another
side, the one that loves reading and writing. She likes to spend
time by herself, to escape to her own world. She wants to have
her own private space. She wants to be the first published seven-
year-old writer. She is building her parallel universe with Harry
Potter. She invents side stories to it. But her favorite book is the
giant *Animal Facts Book*.

Animal remedies usually have two polarities.

– When she was two-and-a-half weeks old she spent forty-eight
hours in the hospital. She had a high fever, so they did a spinal
tap, had IV. She was very upset, hard to calm down. The doctors
feared meningitis so that was the procedure they did. Lucy learned
fear that time. I felt it was the loss of her innocence. She was
very easily startled, cried a lot. There was a tightness, a
guardedness to her. Her whole being showed the fear: what's
going to happen to me? She had a few occasions when she got
very sick. When she was three she got a really bad flu. She had
diarrhea and turned blue from quick dehydration. But she is the
healthiest of my kids! When she feels not all right, she just lies

down and wakes up healthy the next morning. There are these strong polarities in her!

She is truly loyal, devoted. A good example of this is when our neighbors got a puppy: she begged me to accompany them to obedience school. But when they came back after the first visit she saw that her brother also wanted to go. It made her sad; seeing her brother being upset spoiled her happiness. She wanted to find ways that he could go with them next time. She does not want anybody to get hurt or left out. She makes the point to include everybody.

She does not want to kill animals. She says that God is in all animals. One Christmas she got a children's Bible from her grandmother. In that book she saw pictures of the crucifixion. She got so upset that she did not want to be in the same room with the book! She developed a fear of that book. For her, the worst part of it was the nails in Jesus' hand. If someone is hurt or upset it affects her greatly. She is truly empathetic. This shows in her relationship to people and animals as well.

She does not easily freak out, does not lose it. She is tough! Once a friend said she didn't want to play with her. Lucy did not get hurt but rather said: "I will win her back!" She also has a strong sense of justice. If something is not fair she will not be afraid to say it; she will stand up for others as well. She will mediate between the arguing parties. She definitely does not want the shorter stick for herself. She must make sure she gets a good deal.

> This concludes my interview with Lucy's mother. Now Lucy comes in and her mom takes a back seat as Lucy spills the beans. She is eager to talk, answers most questions matter of factly but full of details. She keeps moving around in the wicker chair and often pulls out strings of the rattan.

— *Tell me about your eczema. What is the worst thing about it?*
— It stings in a funny way.

> She pauses, so I ask her again to tell me more about it.

— It is annoying.

As she stops again I keep looking at her encouragingly, waiting for more words to come.

– It stops me from doing things I want to do.

She stops again. This is the point where Lucy's energy starts leading the interview. She tells me her eczema was stopping her from doing things that she liked to do. Once we understand what it is that she likes to do and how the eczema stops her, we will have solved the case. We are at the foot of the mountain that we will climb together with her. We will take her hand and let her lead us to the top.

– I never want to stop writing for anything.
– *Tell me about writing.*
– I use my imagination when I write. I like writing magical stories.

I suddenly realize that she put emphasis on the writing, not so much on inventing these stories.

– *Tell me more about writing these stories.*

Even with the best intentions we often dismiss important information based on our assumptions. When we are looking for images in a child's imagination but they talk about the actual act of writing, it is important to follow their lead and not stick to our original plan of finding out about what they are writing.

– It is an exercise for my hand instead of an exercise for my throat that I do all the time when I talk.
– *Tell me more about exercising your hands.*
– If I am not moving my hands I feel as if they could not move. I also don't like when people keep asking about my eczema. Is it chickenpox? It gets annoying.
– *What do you say?*
– I tell them the truth, but they keep asking. They do it all the time. I have to answer the same question over and over again.
– *What do you mean by annoying?*

– It is boring, saying the same thing again and again.

– *How does it feel when something is boring, when you have to say the same thing again and again?*

– It feels like I should not be doing that. I need to be doing something else but I cannot find out what. That's boring.

> Step by step I am taking her deeper into her own consciousness by asking about her own words. I have no idea where she is going but I know the answer is there, within Lucy. Since she does not know either where we are going, she needs me as a guide to point out the words that she can explain, and by explaining she will unfold some more words that are meaningful for her. This way, listening to all her words and asking about the ones she used with emphasis or the ones I know express deeper layers, lead us together into the realm of her inner expression, the level of sensation.

– *What do you like doing that is not boring?*

– Reading. Fiction is the best. I like reading made-up things. When you can use your imagination. I also like to read facts about animals. I like books about animals.

– *What do you like about those books?*

– I like animals so I like finding out about them.

– *What do you like about reading those books?*

– I want to have animals. I want to spend time with my favorite animals.

– *How does it feel around your favorite animals?*

– It feels good. I am not sure how to explain it.

– *Tell me about that good feeling.*

– My feelings feel different. I am happy, filled with joy.

– *Can you compare it to anything?*

– I don't think so.

– *What is it that you especially like about animals? Do you have a favorite?*

– Horses are my favorite. I like to read horse books. I believe I know everything about horses. When I am ten I can get a horse, my mom says. I have groomed a horse, rode it a few times. Once

we went to a horse farm. I got to ride my favorite horse there.
– *How did you pick which one was your favorite?*
– The way they were with me. I think she liked me.
– *How do you know?*
– When I came over to her stall window she normally came to greet me.

> After discussing her experience with that horse I ask about her dreams to see if the same themes come up there.

– I remember one dream. I was riding on a horse. I got kicked off and landed on another horse. They started playing soccer and I was the ball they were bouncing around!
– *Tell me about the experience in the dream.*
– It was fun flying through the air. I thought that is how it felt to be a bird.

> The important aspect of the dream is the flying through the air. Different people having a similar dream would pick other aspects as meaningful for them. The aspect she picks will lead us further into her inner sensation, her inner experience. So I ask her more about flying through the air.

– Birds have fun flying. They are the leaders; they lead everyone because they are the highest. It is also scary to fall onto the ground. But in the dream I do not fall on the ground but on the back of the horse.

> Another area of children's imagination is what they express in their drawing and painting. I ask about that.

– I like drawing animals and castles. When I draw castles I imagine that I am the queen. The queen is the proud leader. At the same time she is also a knight. She goes to fight but does not kill the enemy. She just makes sure they surrender. She does not want to hurt them.

> I ask Lucy to tell me the story she makes up about this castle and the queen but she says she cannot really

remember. She makes up many stories, many details, but if she does not write them down she forgets them.

— *Why do you like horses so much?*

— I was born liking horses.

> When someone mentions a substance – be it mineral, plant or animal – we do not assume they need the remedy made of that substance. Lucy mentions horses a few times during her interview. The way she describes a horse gives clues to the qualities of the remedy she actually needs. Lucy sees reality in a certain way. She is fascinated with horses for a reason, so I have to find out what the reason is. It will be seen through the qualities of the horse that she recalls.

— The horse has a smooth coat. It is fast: it can run 45 miles per hour. But it is nothing compared to a bird. A special bird.

> She lowers her voice to a mystical whisper.

— It is called the peregrine falcon. The peregrine falcon can fly 220 miles per hour. When it sees a prey it dives with that speed! Peregrine falcons are birds of prey. They are fast, speedy. They dive in the air to catch their prey. They see their prey from great distances. Their eyesight is perfect, like mine. I am not a bit near-sighted. My eyes can act like microscopes. I can see the dust in the sunlight. It looks like tiny bits of hair floating around. I can also see footprints on the moon.

> At this point she is getting tired and informs me that she would love to go outside and do some cartwheels on the grass. I agree as I feel that she has helped me to complete the picture. Our interview ends.

FINDING THE MATCHING REMEDY

When I look at Lucy's case I see a little girl trying to ignore her eczema because it stops her from other things she likes doing. In her fantasy she is a powerful queen who fights like a knight.

She loves her freedom to do her activities. She makes sure that everybody abides by the law, including herself. She makes sure her parents don't drive over the posted limit. As the most powerful fighting queen she will not "kill." She will make the enemy surrender. She includes everybody fairly in her game and reminds others to do so, too.

She loves animals and her connection to them is quite obvious. Animals play an important role in her life. Beside this fact there are more characteristics of the animal kingdom in her symptomatology. Her need to win and her view of competition matches the main characteristic of the animal kingdom.

Within the kingdom we see several characteristics of the subkingdom of birds. People who need bird remedies love freedom. Their spirit soars and flies above the constricting reality of life. They might act in a similar fashion to people who need mineral remedies, but their inner experience will be different: the "mineral person" might experience their climbing of the corporate ladder as duties of responsibility, overcoming obstacles and performing to their standards. In the case of a bird remedy the person will experience it as soaring high in freedom. They are going to strive toward that height as a means to reach the sky, which for them means freedom. These will be the words they are going to use to describe their experience.

Birds also have strong empathy, forming connections to one another through feeling. We saw this in Lucy not wanting her brother to be unhappy and her including everybody in their play.

Fine-tuning our choice for a bird remedy, we find specifically Falcon characteristics in the case. One of the main themes in Falcon cases is speed. It needs no explanation – this comes from the physical characteristic of the bird itself, and this was how Lucy introduced the falcon into our conversation as well.

The core idea in the Falcon remedy is the powerful will. While all bird remedies long for freedom, this idea surfaces most vividly in Falcon. Falcon is made of a remedy of a bird that is kept captive and at the very core of its existence there is the dilemma of following its owner's orders or fly free.

Peregrine falcons are known for their use in falconry. They are the fastest animals in the air. This trait, combined with an obedient nature, make them the perfect match for humans, who learned to train these birds of prey to help them hunt. Falcons are raptors; they have superb vision so they can see prey at great distances. Lucy also says that she has great eyesight with "microscopic vision."

One of Lucy's most intriguing personality traits is her ability to stand up for herself in a way that she feels is fair. She wants to be fair with everybody and make sure that she does not get the shorter stick in the process. Her important issue is that her brother will not surpass her in anything, though it is a tough call because he is not only older but has many talents himself. Lucy is not concerned with pretty clothes and small talk. Rather, she is committed to completing her projects and is concerned with issues that really matter to her. Given that she is only seven years old, that is rather impressive. Other details, such as her empathy toward people and animals, the need to exercise her hands because otherwise they feel paralyzed, or her imagining she is a queen, are part of the experience of people who have benefited from this remedy.

"The Falcon is also known for a desire for the good opinion of others. The image of the falcon on the gloved hand of the falconer, tethered, yet free, is a striking metaphor of this aspect."[8] This is a feature that distinguishes the falcon from other birds: it is captive yet free. It soars and hunts yet it's dominated by the hunter. Lucy's mom says, "She is rebellious at the same time as she is conscientious." It's interesting to note that Lucy's imagery matches that of George's at some points. She, too, talks about the bird as the leader, about the proud queen living in a castle,

---

[8] Shore, Jonathan, M. D, Schriebman, Judy, Hogeland, Anneke, *Birds. Homeopathic Remedies from the Avian Realm*. Berkeley, CA: Homeopathy West (2004) p. 113.

just as George was fascinated with castles and imagined times of the past – of fast-riding horses and hunts.

This is how the fine-tuning process of the remedy hunt happens. First we hear the words describing a large group, the kingdom, then the subkingdom and eventually the specific source of the remedy. That is the energetic essence of the source. In a person there is a certain energetic imbalance with a core pattern. Once we find the energetic essence from a substance that matches the core pattern of the imbalance in the person, we have found the remedy. For Lucy, that remedy is Falcon peregrine. The remedy has the potential to heal. By administering this remedy, the energy of imbalance and illness can be turned into creativity and freedom. When freedom from the ill energy is achieved, the spirit can soar and the patient can be cured.

As mentioned in the Technetium case, when the chief complaint is a skin condition I tend to start treatment with a lower potency in order not to aggravate the skin. This is what happens with Lucy: At her first follow-up her mother reports she has not seen much change.

– The only notable thing was that Lucy talked about a dream she had: We were playing in the woods and a plane crashed near us. We were building a shed, making food out of berries, a cereal. The plane was flying from North Carolina, where I was from in the dream, to Montana. It crashed in Maine.

At this point I give Lucy a dose of Falcon 1M, a higher potency than the first one. My first prescription seemed to be over-cautious and the remedy did not seem to be strong enough. As there has been no great improvement and I am sure in the remedy, and she reconfirmed it, I decide to try the higher potency.

A month later I receive an email from Lucy's mother requesting another dose. She says the first did seem to make a difference but now she is itching more again. So I let her repeat the remedy.

Two months later the family moves away from my area. They decide to give up their urban dwelling and start an exciting new life on a farm. I see Lucy before they move and she is truly enthusiastic about it. She has been promised a horse once they settle down! I send her off with two vials of the remedy, in two different potencies. I get occasional updates on her and always hear what new animals she is sheltering in their farmhouse.

The last I hear from Lucy's family is in a year time, through an email. The best surprise to me is that it includes a poem by Lucy. Her mother writes:

"When I chose the poem, I remembered that Lucy was talking about the falcon in your office. Your session with her was such a learning experience for me. She is still enamored of falcons and often reminds us of how fast they fly. Her skin is stable and improved. I would say that overall it is the best it has been in years. She began weekly riding lessons last week, and I am just wondering if that will help as well. I just realized I do not even know what the remedy was and how you chose it. I would be very curious!"

Here is Lucy's poem:

Freedom Bird

Free as the wind,
Riding the waves,
The falcon soars.
Nesting in a giant tree,
She flaps her huge wings.
Then she dives,
Super fast.
After a tiny rat,
She catches up in no time,
Having a meal.
Free as the wind,
Riding the waves,
She dips, she turns,
Soaring home.

Epilogue

I hope you have found some thought-provoking ideas in this book and you will decide to read more about homeopathy or you might consider trying it out for the first time or going further with your treatment. If you are a homeopathic practitioner or are training to become one, I hope that our explorations into the uses of the Sensation Method may provide you with more tools and ideas that you might choose to call upon. As I said in the beginning, do not blindly follow and believe what I said on these pages. See if it holds true for you. As Samuel Hahnemann said: "*Aude sapere* – Dare to know"[9]

The work of refining the Sensation Method is under way. What we can learn from the old master, Dr. Hahnemann, who kept revising his work until the very end of his life, is the eagerness to keep looking for the truth, the unwavering determination to refine our skills, knowledge, and understanding of human health and disease. We learn from our own mistakes and stay humble while realizing the great power we are holding in our hands when we are continuing the tradition of healing with homeopathy.

---

[9] Hahnemann, Samuel, *Organon of the Medical Art*. Edited and annotated by Wenda Brewster O'Reilly, Redmond, WA: Birdcage Books (1996) p. xiii.

REFERENCES

Dooley, Timothy, N.D., M.D., *Beyond Flat Earth Medicine*. San Diego, CA: Timing Publications (1995)

Hahnemann, Samuel, *Organon of the Medical Art*, edited and annotated by Wenda Brewster O'Reilly. Redmond, WA: Birdcage Books, (1996)

Herrick, Nancy, *Animal Mind, Human Voices. Provings of Eight Animal Remedies*. Nevada City, CA: Hahnemann Clinic Publishing (1998)

Herscu, Paul, N.D., *Stramonium, With an Introduction to Analysis using Cycles and Segments*. Amherst, MA: New England School of Homeopathy Press (1996)

Kent, James Tyler., M.D., *Materia Medica of Homoeopathic Remedies*, London: Homoeopathic Book Service, (1989)

Mangialavori, Massimo, *Knowledge, Seduction and Forsakenness*. Matrix

Mangialavori, Massimo, *Remaining In a Safe Environment: The Sea Remedies*. Matrix

Norland, Misha, *Signatures, Miasms, Aids. Spiritual Aspects of Homeopathy*. Abergavenny, U. K.: Yondercott Press (2003)

Scharmer, C. Otto, *Theory U. Leading From the Future as it Emerges*. Cambridge, MA: Sol (2007)

Scholten, Jan, *Homeopathy and the Elements*. Utrecht, The Netherlands: Stichting Alonnissos (1996)

Senge, Peter, Scharmer, C. Otto, Jaworski, Joseph, Flowers, Betty Sue, *Presence. An Exploration of Profound Change in People, Organizations, and Society*. Cambridge, MA: Sol (2004)

Shore, Jonathan, M.D. Schriebman, Judy, Hogeland, Anneke, *Birds. Homeopathic Remedies from the Avian Realm*. Berkeley, CA: Homeopathy West (2004)

Tolle, Eckhart, *The Power of Now. A Guide to Spiritual Enlightenment.* Vancouver: Namaste Publishing (1999)

Tolle, Eckhart, *A New Earth. Awakening to Your Life's Purpose.* Vancouver: Namaste Publishing (2005)

SUGGESTED READING

INTRODUCTORY HOMEOPATHY

Dooley, Timothy, N.D., M.D., *Beyond Flat Earth Medicine.* San Diego, CA: Timing Publications (1995)

Lansky, Amy, *Impossible Cure: The Promise of Homeopathy.* Portola Valley, CA: R.L. Ranch Press (2003)

Reichenberg-Ullman, Judyth, N.D, L.C. S.W., Ullman, Robert, N.D, Luepker, Ian, N.D., *A Drug-Free Approach to Asperger Syndrome and Autism. Homeopathic Care for Exceptional Kids.* Edmonds, WA: Picnic Point Press (2005)

HISTORY OF HOMEOPATHY

Winston, Julian, *The Faces of Homoeopathy.* Tawa, New Zealand: Great Auk Publishing (1999)

SELF-HEALING WITH HOMEOPATHY

Ullman, Robert, N.D, Reichenberg-Ullman, Judyth, N.D., *Homeopathic Self-Care: The Quick and Easy Guide for the Whole Family.* Roseville, CA: Prima Publishing (1997)

DR. SANKARAN'S BOOKS

Sankaran, Rajan, M.D., *The Spirit of Homoeopathy.* Mumbai, India: Homoeopathic Medical Publishers (1991)

Sankaran, Rajan, M.D., *The Substance of Homoeopathy*. Mumbai, India: Homoeopathic Medical Publishers (1994)

Sankaran, Rajan, M.D., *The Soul of Remedies*. Mumbai, India: Homoeopathic Medical Publishers (1997)

Sankaran, Rajan, M.D., *The System of Homoeopathy*. Mumbai, India: Homoeopathic Medical Publishers (2000)

Sankaran, Rajan, M.D., An *Insight into Plants, volume 1–3*. Mumbai, India: Homoeopathic Medical Publishers. (2002, 2007)

Rajan Sankaran, M.D. *The Sensation in Homoeopathy*. Mumbai, India: Homoeopathic Medical Publishers (2004)

Sankaran, Rajan, M.D., *Sankaran's Schema*. Mumbai, India: Homoeopathic Medical Publishers (2005)

Sankaran, Rajan, M.D., *Sensation Refined*. Mumbai, India: Homoeopathic Medical Publishers (2007)

MORE ON THE SENSATION METHOD

Burch, Melissa, CCH, Aikin, Susana, *Dr. Rajan Sankaran's Correspondence Course: Unit 1–4*. Cambridge, MA: Publication Inner Health, (2006)

Burch, Melissa, CCH, Pershouse, Didi, *Vital Expression: A Manual on Homeopathic Casetaking*. Cambridge, MA: Publication Inner Health (2007)

Vervarcke, Anne, *The Charm of Homeopathy: About Life in General and Homeopathy in Particular*. Leuven, Belgium: The White Room (2006)

INDEX

The Periodic Table of the Elements (Homeopathic Arrangement)

1	2	3	4	5	6	7	8	9	10	11	12	13	14	15	16	17	18
H Hydrogen																	**He** Helium
Li Lithium	**Be** Beryllium											**B** Boron	**C** Carbon	**N** Nitrogen	**O** Oxygen	**F** Fluorine	**Ne** Neon
Na Sodium	**Mg** Magnesium											**Al** Aluminium	**Si** Silicon	**P** Phosphorus	**S** Sulfur	**Cl** Chlorine	**Ar** Argon
K Potassium	**Ca** Calcium	**Sc** Scandium	**Ti** Titanium	**V** Vanadium	**Cr** Chromium	**Mn** Manganese	**Fe** Iron	**Co** Cobalt	**Ni** Nickel	**Cu** Copper	**Zn** Zinc	**Ga** Gallium	**Ge** Germanium	**As** Arsenic	**Se** Selenium	**Br** Bromine	**Kr** Krypton
Rb Rubidium	**Sr** Strontium	**Y** Yttrium	**Zr** Zirconium	**Nb** Niobium	**Mo** Molybdenum	**Tc** Technetium	**Ru** Ruthenium	**Rh** Rhodium	**Pd** Palladium	**Ag** Silver	**Cd** Cadmium	**In** Indium	**Sn** Tin	**Sb** Antimony	**Te** Tellurium	**I** Iodine	**Xe** Xenon
Cs Cesium	**Ba** Barium	**La** Lanthanum	**Hf** Hafnium	**Ta** Tantalum	**W** Tungsten	**Re** Rhenium	**Is** Osmium	**Ir** Iridium	**Pt** Platinum	**Au** Gold	**Hg** Mercury	**Tl** Thallium	**Pb** Lead	**Bi** Bismuth	**Po** Polonium	**At** Astatine	**Rn** Radon
Fr Francium	**Ra** Radium	**Ac** Actinium	**Rf** Rutherfordium	**Db** Dubnium	**Sg** Seaborgium	**Bh** Bohrium	**Hs** Hassium	**Mt** Meitnerium									

ABOUT THE AUTHORS

ILDIKO RAN

is a classical homeopath, practicing in Arlington, MA, in the Greater Boston area. Since graduating from the New England School of Homeopathy in 2000, and The School of Homeopathy in Devon, England in 2001, she has been engaged in postgraduate studies with Dr. Rajan Sankaran, exploring the Sensation Method. Ms. Ran has been active teaching and spreading the word on homeopathy encouraging people of all walks of life to get acquainted with this healing modality. Ms. Ran has been an invited speaker at the Cape Cod Homeopathic Study Group, at NPACE, a conference of a nurses' association, and at a Holistic Psychology class at Lesley University in Cambridge, MA. She has been involved with the peer group of practitioners of the Sensation Method in New England and has been active as a supervisor for novice homeopaths. Ms. Ran enjoys her practice and the intimate setting she shares with her clients in her clinic. She consults with children, adults, adolescents, and the elderly. Her apparent compassion to help her clients is appreciated by many and her enthusiasm for the cutting-edge method of the Sensation Method has born some fruitful accomplishments. Ms. Ran is fluent in English, Russian, Hungarian, and Hebrew. She lives with her husband and five children in Arlington, MA.

ANNA MENYHÉRT

is a writer, editor, university professor, living with her husband and son in Budapest, Hungary. She is currently a freelance writer and studying homeopathy. She received her PhD in literary theory in 2002. Ms. Menyhért worked as an assistant professor of literature at Miskolc University, and later was the head of the department of Hungarology Studies at Balassi Bálint Cultural Institute in Budapest. For six years she was the president of József Attila Circle Literary Union of Young Writers. She has been the vice-president of the European Writers' Congress, an international umbrella organization for two years. She has published two books of essays and criticism, and working on the third, as well as her first book of poetry.

Ms. Menyhért started studying homeopathy two years ago. She finished the introductory courses of the Hungarian Homeopathic Medical Association, participates in the work of the Homeopathic Healing Art Society, taking courses in the Sycosis School of Homeopathy, among them the three-year-course of Dr. Farokh Master, and enrolled at the international home study programme of The School of Homeopathy in Devon, England. Ms. Menyhért has been working under the supervision of Ms. Ran.